Collaborative Insights

Interdisciplinary Perspectives on Musical Care Throughout the Life Course

Edited by

Neta Spiro and Katie Rose M. Sanfilippo

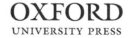

OXFORD
UNIVERSITY PRESS

OXFORD
UNIVERSITY PRESS

Oxford University Press is a department of the University of Oxford. It furthers
the University's objective of excellence in research, scholarship, and education
by publishing worldwide. Oxford is a registered trade mark of Oxford University
Press in the UK and certain other countries.

Published in the United States of America by Oxford University Press
198 Madison Avenue, New York, NY 10016, United States of America.

Library of Congress Control Number: 2022904411

ISBN 978–0–19–753502–8 (pbk.)
ISBN 978–0–19–753501–1 (hbk.)

DOI: 10.1093/oso/9780197535011.001.0001

1 3 5 7 9 8 6 4 2

Paperback printed by LSC Communications, United States of America
Hardback printed by Bridgeport National Bindery, Inc., United States of America

Collaborative Insights

Contents

Acknowledgements

The idea for this book began as a response to questions we had often discussed. Could we provide a brief introduction about music in different care contexts? Could we bring experts from different disciplines to the multifaceted world of music with its different roles in care? Could we seek an understanding of the vast range of music engagement in care contexts throughout the life course while not sacrificing details? We landed on a brief, edited book, bringing together authors from different disciplines for each chapter to explore this work throughout the life course. We also landed on a new term—musical care—to describe the role of music, music listening as well as music-making, in supporting any aspect of people's developmental or health needs: for example, physical and mental health, cognitive and behavioural development, and interpersonal relationships.

Each chapter in the book has been reviewed by two external reviewers, one working as a practitioner-researcher in music therapy and one in a related discipline: Cornelia Bent, Elizabeth Coombes, Philippa Derrington, Claire Flower, Jenny Groarke, Beatriz Ilari, Alexandra Lamont, Raymond MacDonald, Helen Odell-Miller, Rosie Perkins, Jessica Phillips-Silver, and Emma Windle. We would like to thank these esteemed colleagues for generously giving their time and insights. We would also like to thank Michael Schober, Aaron Williamon, Vivette Glover, and Lauren Stewart for providing their valuable insight and support.

Many thanks go to Nordoff Robbins Music Therapy in London, where work on this book began. Many thanks also got to the staff at Oxford University Press, where, in addition to Suzanne Ryan, who enthusiastically received the idea of the book, we thank Sean Decker, Norman Hirschy, the copy editors, and the anonymous reviewers who provided their wholehearted support for publication of the book.

Neta Spiro
Katie Rose M. Sanfilippo
September 2021

Contributors

Stephen Clift, BA, PhD, PFRSPH, is Professor Emeritus, Canterbury Christ Church University, and former Director of the Sidney De Haan Research Centre for Arts and Health. He is a Professorial Fellow of the Royal Society for Public Health (RSPH) and is also Visiting Professor in the International Centre for Community Music, York St John University. Stephen has worked in the field of health promotion and public health for over thirty years, and has made contributions to research, practice and training on HIV/AIDS prevention, sex education, international travel, and health and the health promoting school in Europe. Since 2000 he has pursued research in arts and health and particularly the potential value of group singing for health and well-being. Stephen was one of the founding editors of the journal *Arts & Health: An International Journal for Research, Policy and Practice*.

Ian Cross is Emeritus Professor and Director of the Centre for Music and Science in the Faculty of Music at the University of Cambridge and a Fellow of Wolfson College in the United Kingdom. His early work helped set the agenda for the study of music cognition; he has since published widely in music and science, his work ranging across psychoacoustics, experimental archaeology, neuroscience, evolutionary theory, and clinical applications of music. He is currently investigating whether common processes underpin music and speech as interactive media. He is Editor-in-Chief of SAGE's Open Access journal *Music & Science* and is a classical guitarist.

Shannon de l'Etoile, PhD, is Associate Dean of Graduate Studies and Professor of Music Therapy at the University of Miami, Frost School of Music. Previously, she taught music therapy at the University of Iowa and at Colorado State University (CSU), where she was also a research associate for the Center for Biomedical Research in Music. Her research explores infant response to music, including infant-directed singing in typical and clinical populations, as well as infant movement response to auditory rhythm.

Tia DeNora is Professor of Sociology of Music and Director of Research, in the Department of Sociology/Philosophy at the University of Exeter, UK. She has been a Fellow of the Yale Center for Cultural Sociology since 2004 and is a Fellow of the British Academy. Tia works as a music sociologist, mostly focused on health and well-being. She works in the area of sociological theory but is very committed to empirical research and to the values of 'gentle empiricism' and 'slow' sociology. With Gary Ansdell, she is currently co-editing the Routledge Series *Music & Change: Ecological Perspectives*.

Tamsin Dives studied music therapy in 2005 after a long career as a professional opera singer. Latterly, her work has been based at Christopher's Hospice, more recently managing the Arts team there. Much of the work involved facilitating creative projects between patients at the hospice and other organizations. At the hospice she established a large community choir and a monthly professional concert series. She also helped create an annual conference for art therapists and artists working in the field of palliative care. She has written chapters with a focus on end-of-life care and the final stages of dementia.

Nicola Dunbar completed her Master's in Music Therapy at Nordoff Robbins London Centre, UK, in 2001. Since then, she has worked as a music therapist in schools, nurseries, and a music therapy clinic with children, adolescents, and their parents and carers. Nicola has also worked in adult and elderly mental health settings. She recently trained as a child and family psychotherapist.

Camilla Farrant, MA (Cantab), MMT-NR, Dip.ABRSM, is Head Music Therapist and founder of the Music Therapy Tree in the United Kingdom, an organization that specializes in providing music therapy to children in schools with autism, learning disabilities, and Emotional and Behavioural Disorders, and provides choir projects to vulnerable communities. She read music at Christ's College, Cambridge University, followed by a Master's in Music Therapy at Nordoff Robbins. She worked as a researcher at the Nordoff Robbins London Centre and on projects with Cambridge University's Department of Music and Science. Camilla has authored articles and research papers on music therapy, empathy, and musical interaction, and two specialist books on research evaluation and ethics.

Jo Hockley, OBE, PhD, MSc, RN, is a senior research fellow in the Primary Palliative Care Research Group at the Usher Institute, University of Edinburgh, UK. Jo's career as a nurse specialist in palliative care started at St Christopher's Hospice in 1978, where she embraced the importance of holistic care involving the arts. She has worked across different palliative care settings. She set up the Care Home Project Team at St Christopher's Hospice, London (2008–2013) and has returned to Edinburgh with the vision for a teaching/research-based care home centre (ToRCH) for southeast Scotland.

Katrina Skewes McFerran is Professor and Head of Creative Arts Therapy at the University of Melbourne. Her research has focused on music and adolescents, exploring the potential of music therapy to foster resilience through a series of investigations in the fields of mental health, chronic illness, and disability. She has also investigated music listening by adolescents, particularly focusing on variations in uses of music that are linked to mental health. She has published two books on these topics: *Adolescents, Music and Music Therapy* and *Building Music Cultures in Schools* and has co-authored the second edition of *Receptive Music Therapy*.

Simon Procter, PhD, is Director of Music Services (Education, Research and Public Affairs) at Nordoff Robbins, London, UK. Simon trained as a music therapist with Nordoff Robbins in London and has since worked primarily within adult mental health services, as well as in the training of music therapists. He has oversight of Nordoff Robbins' education and research activities as well as being active in communicating about their work in the public sphere. Simon as a researcher is primarily an ethnographer, passionate about learning from people's expertise and experiences.

Tal-Chen Rabinowitch is an Assistant Professor at the School of Creative Arts Therapies at the University of Haifa, Israel, where she heads the Music and Social Development Lab. She is interested in understanding the role music plays in children's social and emotional development and the cognitive mechanisms that underlie it. Tal-Chen earned a PhD in Music at the Centre for Music and Science, University of Cambridge, UK, followed by postdoctoral work at the Hebrew University of Jerusalem, and at the University of Washington, Seattle, USA.

Suvi Saarikallio is Associate Professor of Music Education, Docent of Psychology, and currently the Vice-Head (Head of Research) of the Department of Music, Art and Culture studies at University of Jyväskylä, Finland. Her research addresses music in youth development, emotion regulation, and well-being, bridging the fields of music psychology, music education, and music therapy. Suvi is a co-editor of the *Handbook of Music, Adolescents, and Wellbeing* and currently the President of Finnish Society for Music Education (FiSME) and the Vice-President of European Society for the Cognitive Sciences of Music (ESCOM).

Katie Rose M. Sanfilippo is currently a research fellow in the Centre for Healthcare Innovation Research at City, University of London. She was previously a postdoctoral fellow in psychology at Goldsmiths, University of London where she also received her PhD. She is also an affiliated lecturer in music at University of Cambridge. Her current research is exploring the application of music-based interventions to support maternal mental health across different cultural contexts in Africa and the United Kingdom. She has worked with various policymakers, charities, and health organizations to promote maternal mental health in educational and health policy agendas. She worked for two years as a research assistant in the research team at Nordoff Robbins Music Therapy Charity.

Neta Spiro is Reader in Performance Science at the Royal College of Music and an honorary Research Fellow at Imperial College London. She was previously Research Fellow at Royal Holloway, University of London, and at the New School for Social Research, New York, and Head of Research at Nordoff Robbins, London. Neta taught at the Faculty of Music, University of Cambridge, where she continues as an honorary member. Two questions underlie her research: What is the potential role of music in people's health and well-being, and what is communicated when we make music together?

Sandra E. Trehub, PhD, a retired Professor of Psychology at the University of Toronto, Canada, has published extensively on music perception and on the role on music in the lives of infants and young children. Her scholarly honours include a Lifetime Achievement Award from the Society for Music Perception and Cognition (USA). Currently she chairs the board of *St. James Town Community Arts*, a charitable organization that provides free music and arts instruction for underserved children in Toronto.

Giorgos Tsiris, PhD, is senior lecturer in music therapy at Queen Margaret University and arts lead at St Columba's Hospice Care in Edinburgh, UK. He has worked in diverse palliative care contexts and led award-winning initiatives building musical communities and disrupting societal assumptions about death and dying. Giorgos is the founding editor of *Approaches: An Interdisciplinary Journal of Music Therapy*, and his work has been published widely to include two books on service evaluation and research ethics, respectively, for arts therapists and arts in health practitioners. His research areas include spirituality, end-of-life care, and evaluation.

Stuart Wood, PhD, is a music therapist and an independent scholar of Music & Health. His work encompasses music therapy, community music and medical humanities, embracing arts-based, practice-based and ethnographic methodologies. He is a Research Associate with the Alzheimer's Scotland Centre for Policy and Practice at the University of West of Scotland, and a doctoral supervisor at the Guildhall School of Music and Drama in London. His published works and international lectures address topics such as music and dementia, participatory research methods, and communal approaches to music therapy. He was awarded an MBE in 2017 for Services to Music Therapy and Care.

Introduction

Interdisciplinary perspectives on musical care throughout the life course

Katie Rose M. Sanfilippo and Neta Spiro

Music can provide care for people throughout their lives, responding to people's health, educational, and social needs. Music is multifaceted in its nature. It is ubiquitous, emotional, ambiguous, and social (MacDonald et al., 2012). It moves through different contexts, from clinical, to educational, to everyday settings (MacDonald, 2013). The recognition of the multifaceted and complex nature of music within care settings has resulted in calls for more interdisciplinary understanding of how and why music can provide care (Heydon et al., 2020; MacDonald et al., 2012; Tsiris et al., 2016). In response to these calls, this book aims to provide interdisciplinary insight into how musical care is understood and provided during different stages of the life course. It does so by bringing together music practitioners and researchers to collaboratively write each chapter. Each chapter covers one period during the life course, discusses musical care from an interdisciplinary perspective, and offers directions for future work. The life course structure highlights the connections and themes present in approach, context, and musical care practices throughout our lives and the call for future interdisciplinary work paves the way for new endeavours. Rather than a thorough account of research in musical care in general, this book illustrates the wealth of understanding that can be gained from interdisciplinary collaboration by presenting snippets of the state of the art in musical care throughout the life course.

In recent years, there has been a growth of interest in the field of music and health, as indicated by books on music psychology, music therapy, and music education (Cross et al., 2008; Edwards, 2016; MacDonald, 2013; McPherson & Welch, 2012; Wigram et al., 2013). These books often give thorough overviews of research in the field. They often also bring together numerous disciplines to inform our understanding of musical care, thus indicating the multidisciplinary nature of music in health, education, and care settings. Nevertheless, in such books divides in discipline and methodology often persist with focus on one perspective, be it from music therapy, music education, or music psychology. This book recognizes these disciplinary divides but aims to highlight the bridges and connections between disciplines, methodologies, and understandings.

Katie Rose M. Sanfilippo and Neta Spiro, *Introduction* In: *Collaborative Insights.* Edited by: Neta Spiro and Katie Rose M. Sanfilippo, Oxford University Press. © Oxford University Press 2022. DOI: 10.1093/oso/9780197535011.003.0001

Through our work as researchers we have encountered the need for discussion and collaboration between the different disciplines that surround musical care (Sanfilippo & Spiro, 2017). We have been faced with opportunities and challenges that can be encountered through these types of collaborations. For example, opportunities include the introduction of new methods to explore old questions, while challenges include differences in terminology that lead to difficulties in communication across disciplinary boundaries. We hope that through this book we can shed more light on what these opportunities are and see the results of existing collaborations that have addressed these challenges.

Writing *Collaborative Insights*

This book's co-authored structure and its calls for research illustrate the possibility and importance of interdisciplinary collaboration in musical care. One author of each chapter is a music therapist who brings their knowledge of music therapy theory, practice, and research. For continuity, we have chosen music therapists to represent musical care professionals, a group that also includes community musicians, music and health practitioners, and music educators. This project began at Nordoff Robbins in the United Kingdom, a music therapy charity that provides music therapy services, education, and research. Therefore, several of the music therapist authors are trained in this approach but some have additional training in other approaches and, all of the authors were invited to include research that covers a wide range of music practices. The other author for each chapter is a researcher with work in a related discipline. These related disciplines include psychology, education, sociology, and public health. Two chapters—Musical care in adolescence and Musical care in adulthood— capitalize on an existing interdisciplinary collaborations between music therapists and researchers and one chapter—Musical care at the end of life—grows from an existing collaboration that also includes a medical practitioner.

Working towards the aim of creating a truly interdisciplinary and cohesive book, authors and editors collaborated throughout the writing process. A workshop brought the authors and editors together to discuss their plans. Authors shared their chapter drafts with one another, allowing editors and authors to find connections and differences in order to create a cohesive journey for the reader. The chapters lead to proposed research avenues that invite readers to engage in future interdisciplinary thinking, practice, and research. All authors could contribute to these ideas, giving different perspectives on future directions and questions. In summary, through collaborative action, this book presents examples and future directions of musical care throughout the life course.

Musical care

We define the term musical care as the role of music—music listening as well as music-making—in supporting any aspect of people's developmental or health needs: for example, physical and mental health, cognitive and behavioural development, and interpersonal relationships. The term musical care can be applied and be made more specific in particular contexts. For example, in this book each group of chapter authors adopts the term musical care in a way that is more specific to their chapter. The flexible adoption of the term throughout this book illustrates its wide scope of applicability, reflecting the far-reaching and evolving nature of music practices and their applications within care. Therefore, the term musical care invites the blurring of boundaries across different areas of expertise, as well as across musical care activities, their roles, and the contexts in which they happen.

Blurred boundaries

Numerous areas of expertise, be they professional, disciplinary, from practice, or from personal experience, are relevant to musical care. Examples include, medical professions, music psychology research disciplines, music therapy practice, and people's lived experiences. The boundaries between these areas of expertise are sometimes necessary and productive but can also be limiting and challenging (Liberati et al., 2016; Sims et al., 2015). Musical care's wide scope and broad definition can allow for the blurred boundaries between these areas of expertise to be acknowledged and explored further.

There are many ways in which musical care activities play a role in therapeutic, health, educational, everyday, and community contexts (MacDonald, 2013): from music therapy with children with autism spectrum disorders to help with joint attention (e.g., Kim et al., 2008), to music listening interventions to reduce preoperative anxiety (e.g., Bradt et al., 2013); from music teaching associated with improved social and cognitive skills in children (e.g., Hallam, 2010), to personal everyday music listening for emotion regulation (e.g., Sloboda & O'Neill, 2001), and to community choirs that can support psychological well-being (e.g., Clift et al., 2010). Despite the distinctiveness of these different musical care activities, as well as their roles and contexts, there can be striking similarities between them (MacDonald, 2013). Understanding the boundaries that often exist within musical care is relevant. However, equally relevant is the acknowledgement of where those boundaries are blurred. This blurring is important for future development and understanding of musical care.

Music in musical care

What music sounds like in musical care, who and how many people it includes, where it takes place, and its purpose can be different and wide ranging (e.g., Clarke et al., 2012; DeNora, 2000; Small, 1999). How music sounds and what instruments are playing are defined by the community engaging in that musical care activity (Cross,

2001). Music can be improvised like in a music therapy session or scripted like in a hit song performed by a community choir, or a combination of the two. These elements sit on an ever-shifting spectrum that includes different types of sounds and structures simultaneously.

The music in musical care involves participants with a range of expertise from the more musically experienced to the less. It also involves a range of specialists, such as music therapists or choir conductors. It can also involve being alone or part of a dyad, a small group or a large group. For example, someone could write songs on their own, participate in a one-to-one music therapy session, or sing in a community choir. In each experience of music in musical care, participants can take on different (and sometimes varying) roles. For example, participants can listen or play, lead or follow, observe or co-create, and can shift between these roles.

The music in musical care can happen in private and public places—in one-to-one therapy in a private room or in a communal space in a care home. It is often associated with formal settings, such as hospitals or schools, but can happen informally when, for example, parents sing with their infants or we listen to music privately. By using the term musical care, we prioritize the connections among these diverse musical activities.

The boundaries between activities that can be seen as having care elements and those that do not are blurred. One recurring fundamental question about the purpose of music within our lives concerns a tension between music engagement for its own sake and a utilitarian view of music (Scherer & Zentner, 2008; Winner et al., 2013). For some, the purpose of engaging in music can be mainly aesthetic (e.g., Aigen, 2007; Mark, 1982); for others it can have a function beyond the engagement itself (e.g., Hanson-Abromeit, 2015; Hargreaves & North, 1999; Maloney, 2017; Schäfer et al., 2013). In our view, the boundaries between these purposes of musical engagement are blurred. Whether implicitly or explicitly acknowledged, the purpose of music within musical care can be both aesthetic and functional.

Life course

Musical care happens throughout the life course, from the prenatal stage to the end of life. Each chapter of this book focuses on one life stage. Segmenting according to life stages is common in disciplines such as developmental psychology (e.g., Lally & Valentine-French, 2017) and sociology (e.g., Clair et al., 1993) as a way to interpret people's everyday experiences and realities (Holstein & Gubrium, 2007).

Scholars have acknowledged that the life course and its stages are socially constructed (Holstein & Gubrium, 2007; Kohli & Meyer, 1986), and culturally and personally experienced and acknowledged. The meaning of these experiences is shaped across and within different times during our lives (Clausen, 1985; Holstein & Gubrium, 2007). Sociologists, from the constructionist perspective, examine the way in which meaning is constructed *through* or *across* the life course in general. They focus on stages (such as adolescence) as well as transitions between them (such as from adolescence to adulthood). Another, more constitutive approach examines how the life course is used as an interpretative *resource*; how it is used as a way for people to make sense of their life experiences through time. For example, age-related expectations of an adolescent may be used to discuss whether particular behaviours can be expected or not (see Holstein & Gubrium, 2007). Within this book we take on both the constructionist and constitutive perspectives to look at how people experience musical care both through and across the life course and use the chapter structure as an interpretative resource to describe experiences often documented in each life stage.

These divisions of the life course, though a helpful resource, lead to prioritization of particular stages in our understanding of musical care in practice and research. For example, we chose to divide the book into six life stages. However, put perhaps simplistically, the number of years accounted for in the different chapters can be markedly different: infancy covers around 3 years of life, while adulthood covers many multiples of this duration. Indeed, these age-related categories could have been divided further (e.g., with more fine-grained distinctions in the adulthood life stage or indeed infancy). Similarly, we place the chapter on the end of life as a separate stage chronologically at the end of the book, though of course life can end during any stage. Even with these limitations, through the connections we draw across the chapters and those we discuss in the Synthesis, we can explore how musical care can transcend these constructed boundaries.

The life stage structure has not been systemically used in discussion of research and practices in the arena of musical care. By using the life stages as our framework, we highlight the transformations and changes in the application of musical care as life progresses. We prioritize the experiences within the life stages over the diagnoses and contexts usually associated with them.

Interdisciplinary collaboration

Collaborations involve different types of relationships between disciplines: multidisciplinary, interdisciplinary, and transdisciplinary (Rosenfield, 1992). Multidisciplinary collaboration involves experts from different disciplines working side by side, drawing on knowledge from one another's disciplines while staying within their own boundaries. Interdisciplinary collaboration involves interactive work wherein knowledge is explicitly exchanged and integrated, from the inception of a project and throughout (Choi & Pak, 2006). Transdisciplinary collaboration involves the most synthesis between collaborators. Though interdisciplinary research focuses on collaboration based on a common question, transdisciplinary collaboration goes beyond this by, for example, creating a common conceptual framework, and either learning one another's disciplinary language or creating a new common one (Aboelela et al., 2007). This type of collaboration is rarely achieved.

Multidisciplinary collaboration is not unfamiliar or new in musical care. In their daily work, many musical care practitioners are involved in multidisciplinary teams that include, for example, medical practitioners or teachers. Many researchers also work within multidisciplinary teams, often with researchers or practitioners from other disciplines. Even with the frequency of multidisciplinary working, truly interdisciplinary research and practice is less common. An advantage of interdisciplinary thinking and work—with its reciprocal interaction between disciplines—is that working together in this way necessitates blurring of disciplinary boundaries (Choi & Pak, 2006). This type of work and research brings with it opportunities, such as the development of new approaches, as well as challenges and hurdles such as differences in assumptions of what is important or interesting, what counts as trustworthy, and what words mean (Spiro & Schober, 2014; Tsiris et al., 2016).

As musical care and the life course are each such broad and multifaceted concepts, interdisciplinary collaboration is particularly fitting. This type of collaboration within musical care helps address the biases and limitations of individual disciplines' understandings, methodologies, and expertise. Both researchers and practitioners sometimes have to adapt their thinking and methods on the basis of what they find in one another's work. For example, agreement needs to be reached about what constitutes helpful data, how best to analyse it, or what can be taken as convincing evidence. Though multidisciplinary publications and research are common in this field, truly interdisciplinary research, involving collaboration from inception to implementation, is less common and more difficult to identify on the basis of how research is discussed, published, and indexed.

Therefore, rather than focusing on previously published interdisciplinary work, this book prioritizes interdisciplinary perspectives on research and practice in musical care throughout the life course. In this book the authors bring together research from a wide range of disciplines and interpret it from their combined complementary disciplinary viewpoints, leading to collectively reached new insights. Interdisciplinary thinking from inception was facilitated through an opening seminar with all authors. Interdisciplinarity is woven into this book through the collaboration of authors from different disciplines in each chapter. The authors make transparent the tensions and opportunities that can arise in interdisciplinary work. At the end of each chapter the authors lay out possible interdisciplinary avenues for research and these ideas are brought together in the final chapter, the Synthesis, to chart possible interdisciplinary paths forward within musical care.

Chapter summaries

This is the first book that takes an explicit interdisciplinary perspective on musical care throughout the life course. Each of the book's chapters focuses on examples from different life stages, beginning with infancy and carrying through to the end of life. Each chapter works to ensure there is an integration of research and practice. Some chapter authors also include explicit case studies from their work as practitioners. Across the six different chapters, aspects and themes of musical care are brought to the fore, while others fade into the background, perhaps to return later. The book's representation of the ebb and flow of the uses and effects of musical care throughout the life course gives a broader understanding of musical care.

In Chapter 1 Katie Rose Sanfilippo, Shannon de l'Etoile, and Sandra Trehub discuss two types of musical care in infancy. Natural musical care refers to everyday uses of music in interactions with infants, reinforcing cultural practices. Targeted musical care draws on educational and clinical approaches to create musical interventions and music therapy practices. The chapter leads to three conclusions about musical care in infancy. First, infants are motivated music listeners who engage with and learn from music in their daily lives. Second, musical caregiving rituals, involving singing to infants, occur in every known culture and have beneficial consequences for the infant and caregiver. Finally, targeted musical care can support infants and caregivers in the context of various challenges.

In Chapter 2 Camilla Farrant, Tal-Chen Rabinowitch, and Nicola Dunbar focus on drawing together research and clinical perspectives in three main areas of childhood development: cognitive, physiological/physical, and social-emotional development. They identify three modes of musical engagement: music listening, music learning, and musical interaction with others. They conclude that music is an act of caregiving that can influence the quality of a child's development.

In Chapter 3 Suvi Saarikallio and Katrina Skewes McFerran focus on work from their long-standing collaboration as a music psychologist and a music therapist. They discuss musical care for emotional development and self-regulation in adolescence. They also discuss musical care in personal and social identity. In doing so they discuss music as an expression, and development, of identity and also as a way to connect. Finally, they explore unhelpful uses of music in adolescence and in response investigate the promotion of more helpful and intentional uses of musical care in adolescence.

In Chapter 4 Simon Procter and Tia DeNora focus on four aspects of musical care in adulthood: self-care, familial or emotional ties, industrialized and commercialized provision, and music therapy and related musical forms of service provision. Taking a cultural sociological approach and integrating music therapy practice experience and expertise, they highlight the musical threads, which can involve very brief moments of interaction, that run through care-based relationships and situations throughout adulthood.

In Chapter 5, Stuart Wood and Stephen Clift explore how musical care can be employed as a strategy of health and social care in older age with individuals, groups, and communities. They discuss research on group singing and music therapy interventions and musical care in the context of nursing. They conclude that musical care may help ensure that older adulthood remains a time of flourishing.

In Chapter 6, Giorgos Tsiris, Jo Hockley, and Tamsin Dives discuss the diverse forms of musical care at the end of life that are characterized by different aims, practices, and contexts. They consider the private-public and specialist-everyday continua of musical care at the end of life and its ability to reach and support people across their health-illness trajectories. They conclude that musical care can offer a sense of well-being and promote quality of life for the dying person and those around them. It can generate a sense of individual as well as communal flourishing by encompassing the interconnections between people and their environments.

What to expect

Though we introduced the term musical care as the role of music—music listening as well as music-making—in supporting any aspect of people's developmental or health needs, as you will see, each chapter's authors apply the term in a way that is specific to each life stage. Taken together, these specific applications highlight some ways in which musical care is positioned. For example, the term musical care might be adopted to describe everyday musical interactions or more formal sets of practices or approaches used to support specific needs of individuals or groups. The scope of who is the focus of care shifts throughout the chapters. In infancy and end of life the family unit is specifically targeted. In adolescence, peers come more into view, and in adulthood familial and professional obligations are highlighted, though musical care is often still focused on individuals, even going so far as emphasising self care. The chapters on older adulthood and end of life consider musical care as applicable beyond the individual to include specific health care communities and wider society.

This book aims to blur the boundaries between contexts, disciplines, and outcomes. The chapters show musical care happening in various contexts. For example, in the childhood chapter, educational contexts are drawn out, whereas in older adulthood and end-of-life, hospice and care contexts become a place of focus. In infancy, the neonatal intensive care unit is one context, but the home environment is also investigated. The chapters also draw on a range of disciplines related to practice and academic research. Different disciplines' research and theories dominate or recede in the different chapters, depending on the life stage, the musical care context, and the expertise of the authors.

Taken together, the chapters show the breadth of outcomes in musical care throughout the life course, including physical, psychological, developmental, social, and educational areas of impact. Though some outcomes (e.g., social and physiological) seem to be present throughout the book, some chapters lend themselves to focus more on specific areas of impact. For example, developmental outcomes are highlighted in the infancy and childhood chapters. Physical outcomes come to the fore within the older-age chapter, and educational outcomes do so within the childhood and end-of-life chapters. As the practice of musical care, as well as its associated research aims, applications, and outcomes are so varied, it is important to find a balance between learning from individual differences in experience, evaluation of evidence across many people, and understanding the underlying mechanisms that are fundamental to music's use. Therefore, the chapters in this book address not only if music can provide for people's needs but also how and why it might do so.

These chapters, when sewn together, not only find a balance in representing the distinctive contexts, disciplines, and outcomes specific to each time in a person's life, but also weave together the commonalities that lie across the life course. In so doing, this book blurs boundaries, underlines the breadth of musical care practice and research, and simultaneously points to ways forward.

A call to action

This is not just a reference book but also the start of a conversation and a call to action. The end of each chapter and the Synthesis directly address areas for future research. Whether you are a practitioner interested in musical care, a music psychologist interested in musical care practice and approaches, a music therapist interested in wider research areas, or a student embarking in any discipline represented in this text, we hope that you feel inspired to engage further with interdisciplinary work and perspectives on musical care. We hope this book will be a catalyst for new collaborations that will bring new insights to musical care throughout the life course.

References

Aboelela, S. W., Larson, E., Bakken, S., Carrasquillo, O., Formicola, A., Glied, S. A., Haas, J., & Gebbie, K. M. (2007). Defining interdisciplinary research: Conclusions from a critical review of the literature. *Health Services Research*, 42(1), 329–346. https://doi.org/10.1111/j.1475-6773.2006.00621.x

Aigen, K. (2007). In defense of beauty: A role for the aesthetic in music therapy theory. Part I: The development of aesthetic theory in music therapy. *Nordic Journal of Music Therapy*, 16(2), 112–128. https://doi.org/10.1080/08098130709478181

Bradt, J., Dileo, C., & Shim, M. (2013). Music interventions for preoperative anxiety. *Cochrane Database of Systematic Reviews*, 6. https://doi.org/10.1002/14651858.CD006908.pub2

Choi, B. C., & Pak, A. W. (2006). Multidisciplinarity, interdisciplinarity and transdisciplinarity in health research, services, education and policy: 1. Definitions, objectives, and evidence of effectiveness. *Clinical and Investigative Medicine*, 29(6), 351–364. http://uvsalud.univalle.edu.co/pdf/politica_formativa/documentos_de_estudio_referencia/multidisciplinarity_interdisicplinarity_transdisciplinarity.pdf

Clair, J. M., Karp, D. A., & Yoels, W. C. (1993). *Experiencing the life cycle: A social psychology of aging*. Charles C. Thomas Publisher.

Clarke, E., Dibben, N., & Pitts, S. (2010). *Music and mind in everyday life*. Oxford University Press.

Clausen, J. A. (1985). *The life course: A sociological perspective*. Pearson.

Clift, S., Hancox, G., Morrison, I., Hess, B., Kreutz, G., & Stewart, D. (2010). Choral singing and psychological wellbeing: Quantitative and qualitative findings from English choirs in a cross-national survey. *Journal of Applied Arts & Health*, 1(1), 19–34. https://doi.org/10.1386/jaah.1.1.19/1

Cross, I. (2001). Music, cognition, culture, and evolution. *Annals of the New York Academy of sciences, 930*(1), 28–42. https://doi.org/10.1111/j.1749-6632.2001.tb05723.x

Cross, I., Hallam, S., & Thaut, M. (Eds.). (2008). *The Oxford handbook of music psychology*. Oxford University Press. https://doi.org/10.1093/oxfordhb/9780199298457.001.0001

DeNora, T. (2000). *Music in everyday life*. Cambridge University Press. https://doi.org/10.2307/3384690

Edwards, J. (Ed.). (2016). *The Oxford handbook of music therapy*. Oxford University Press. https://doi.org/10.1093/oxfordhb/9780199639755.001.0001

Hallam, S. (2010). The power of music: Its impact on the intellectual, social and personal development of children and young people. *International Journal of Music Education, 28*(3), 269–289. https://doi.org/10.1177/0255761410370658

Hanson-Abromeit, D. (2015). A conceptual methodology to define the therapeutic function of music. *Music Therapy Perspectives, 33*(1), 25–38. https://doi.org/10.1093/mtp/miu061

Hargreaves, D. J., & North, A. C. (1999). The functions of music in everyday life: Redefining the social in music psychology. *Psychology of Music, 27*(1), 71–83. https://doi.org/10.1177/0305735699271007

Heydon, R., Fancourt, D., & Cohen, A. (Eds.). (2020). *The Routledge companion to interdisciplinary studies in singing. Vol. III. Wellbeing*. Routledge.

Holstein, J. A., & Gubrium, J. F. (2007). Constructionist perspectives on the life course. *Sociology Compass, 1*(1), 335–352. https://doi.org/10.1111/j.1751-9020.2007.00004.x

Kim, J., Wigram, T., & Gold, C. (2008). The effects of improvisational music therapy on joint attention behaviors in autistic children: A randomized controlled study. *Journal of Autism and Developmental Disorders, 38*(9), 1758–1766. https://doi.org/10.1007/s10803-008-0566-6

Kohli, M., & Meyer, J. W. (1986). Social structure and social construction of life stages. *Human Development, 29*(3), 145–149. https://doi.org/10.1159/000273038

Lally, M., & Valentine-French, S. (2017). *Lifespan development: A psychological perspective* (2nd ed.). College of Lake County Foundation.

Liberati, E. G., Gorli, M., & Scaratti, G. (2016). Invisible walls within multidisciplinary teams: Disciplinary boundaries and their effects on integrated care. *Social Science & Medicine, 150*, 31–39. https://doi.org/10.1016/j.socscimed.2015.12.002

MacDonald, R. A. R. (2013). Music, health, and well-being: A review. *International Journal of Qualitative Studies on Health and Well-Being, 8*(1). 20635. https://doi.org/10.3402/qhw.v8i0.20635

MacDonald, R. A. R., Kreutz, G., & Mitchell, L. (Eds.). (2012). *Music, health, and wellbeing*. Oxford University Press. https://doi.org/10.1093/acprof:oso/9780199586974.001.0001

Maloney, L. (2017). Music as water: The functions of music from a utilitarian perspective. *AVANT. Pismo Awangardy Filozoficzno-Naukowej, 8*, 57–67.

Mark, M. L. (1982). The evolution of music education philosophy from utilitarian to aesthetic. *Journal of Research in Music Education, 30*(1), 15–21. https://doi.org/10.2307/3344863

McPherson, G. E., & Welch, G. F. (Eds.). (2012). *The Oxford handbook of music education*. Oxford University Press. https://doi.org/10.1093/oxfordhb/9780199928019.001.0001

Pearce, E., Launay, J., & Dunbar, R. I. M. (2015). The ice-breaker effect: Singing mediates fast social bonding. *The Royal Society Open Science, 2*(10), 150221. https://doi.org/10.1098/rsos.150221

Rosenfield, P. L. (1992). The potential of transdisciplinary research for sustaining and extending linkages between the health and social sciences. *Social Science and Medicine, 35*(11), 1343–1357. https://doi.org/10.1016/0277-9536(92)90038-R

Sanfilippo, K. R. M., & Spiro, N. (2017). The Third Nordoff Robbins Plus Conference 'Exploring music in therapeutic and community settings.' *Approaches: An Interdisciplinary Journal of Music Therapy|, 9*(1), 159–163.

Schäfer, T., Sedlmeier, P., Städtler, C., & Huron, D. (2013). The psychological functions of music listening. *Frontiers in Psychology, 4,* 511. https://doi.org/10.3389/fpsyg.2013.00511

Scherer, K., & Zentner, M. (2008). Music evoked emotions are different—More often aesthetic than utilitarian. *Behavioral and Brain Sciences, 31*(5), 595–596. https://doi.org/10.1017/S0140525X08005505

Sims, S., Hewitt, G., & Harris, R. (2015). Evidence of collaboration, pooling of resources, learning and role blurring in interprofessional healthcare teams: A realist synthesis. *Journal of Interprofessional Care, 29*(1), 20–25. https://doi.org/10.3109/13561820.2014.939745

Sloboda, J. A., & O'Neill, S. A. (2001). Emotions in everyday listening to music. In *Music and emotion: Theory and research* (pp. 415–429). https://doi.org/10.1017/CBO9781107415324.004

Small, C. (1999). Musicking—The meanings of performing and listening: A lecture. *Music Education Research, 1*(1), 9–22. https://doi.org/10.1080/1461380990010102

Spiro, N., & Schober, M. F. (2014). Perspectives on music and communication: An introduction. *Psychology of Music, 42*(6), 771–775. https://doi.org/10.1177/0305735614549493

Tsiris, G., Derrington, P., Sparks, P., Spiro, N., & Wilson, G. (2016). Interdisciplinary dialogues in music, health and wellbeing: Difficulties, challenges and pitfalls. *ISME Commission on Special Education and Music Therapy 2016 Proceedings,* 58–70. https://eresearch.qmu.ac.uk/handle/20.500.12289/4647.

Wigram, T., Saperston, B., & West, R. (2013). *Art & science of music therapy: A handbook.* Routledge.

Williams, E., Dingle, G. A., & Clift, S. (2018). A systematic review of mental health and wellbeing outcomes of group singing for adults with a mental health condition. *European Journal of Public Health, 28*(6), 1035–1042. https://doi.org/10.1093/eurpub/cky115

Winner, E., Goldstein, T. R., & Vincent-Lancrin, S. (2013). *Art for art's sake? The impact of arts education* (Educational Research and Innovation [Ed]). OECD Publishing. https://doi.org/10.1787/9789264180789-en

1
Musical care in infancy

Supporting infants and their caregivers

Katie Rose M. Sanfilippo, Shannon de l'Etoile, and Sandra E. Trehub

Introduction

Developing infants could not survive, let alone thrive, without committed caregivers. As a result, musical care in infancy concerns not only the infant but also the caregiver–infant dyad. Musical engagement is an integral part of the caregiver–infant relationship, with caregivers around the world incorporating singing into their infant care routines. Maternal or caregiver singing in the context of infant care provides a template for musical engagement throughout life and an inspiration for musical care with special populations.

We define musical care in infancy (until about 3 years of age) as the use of music—music listening as well as music-making—to support infant care, parental care, and the dyadic relationship. Musical care in infancy, as construed here, encompasses two broad realms. From psychological and sociological perspectives, *natural* musical care is seen in cultural practices that accommodate infant nurture and development, supporting infant and parental well-being in the context of the caregiving relationship. Emanating from this foundation, *targeted* musical care draws on educational and clinical approaches involving musical interventions and music therapy to enhance outcomes in parents and infants who are at risk of less-than-optimal functioning.

The aims of *natural* and *targeted* musical care may shift over the course of infant development, depending on the needs of the dyad or family. In pregnancy, most musical care aims to enhance the well-being of expectant mothers, but it has the potential for short- as well as long-term benefits for the dyad. Postnatal musical care targets infant needs, parental well-being, and the unique dynamics of the parent–infant dyad and family unit.

The social and emotional consequences of parent–infant musical interactions are garnering increasing attention in several disciplines such as psychology, sociology, ethnomusicology, public health, social work, rehabilitation medicine, and music therapy. The present chapter exemplifies collaboration across some of these disciplines. Katie Rose Sanfilippo, a researcher in psychology, studies music and health, with a focus on participatory music-making (e.g., group singing) to support women's mental health during pregnancy. Shannon de l'Etoile, a professor and practitioner of

Katie Rose M. Sanfilippo, Shannon de l'Etoile, and Sandra E. Trehub, *Musical care in infancy* In: *Collaborative Insights*. Edited by: Neta Spiro and Katie Rose M. Sanfilippo, Oxford University Press. © Oxford University Press 2022. DOI: 10.1093/oso/9780197535011.003.0002 music therapy, studies responsiveness to music in typically developing (TD) infants and those with special needs. Sandra Trehub, a retired professor of psychology, focuses on music perception in infancy as well as the nature and consequences of caregivers' singing to infants.

Contemporary care in pregnancy and infancy is multidisciplinary, involving midwives, arts-in-health practitioners, psychologists, perinatal mental health practitioners, and paediatricians, creating challenges as well as opportunities for merging ideas and skills to optimize musical care. We begin by reviewing research, primarily from developmental psychology, on the capacity for infant musical engagement, prenatally as well as postnatally, which provides the foundation for musical care interventions. We proceed to discuss mothers' (or primary caregivers') intuitive singing and musical care rituals across cultures, incorporating insights from sociology, anthropology, and ethnomusicology that highlight *natural* musical care. In the final part of the chapter, we focus on musical care interventions and music therapy research and practice, or *targeted* musical care, drawing upon music psychology, medical ethnomusicology, perinatal mental health, obstetrics, paediatrics, and music therapy. We consider the role of musical care in supporting maternal physical and mental health, prenatally and postnatally, as well as infant physical and mental health. We describe musical care interventions and music therapy practice for clinical populations, including infants with disabilities and premature infants in the neonatal intensive care unit (NICU). Finally, we discuss the multidisciplinary nature of musical care in infancy and suggest future directions for research and practice.

Infants' musical capacities

Understanding the nature of infants' auditory environment and their responsiveness to sound patterns is crucial for optimizing the selection of musical materials and contexts for *natural* or *targeted* musical interactions. The developing fetus is surrounded by sound, both internal (e.g., maternal heartbeat, digestive sounds, vocalizations) and external (e.g., speech, music) (Lecanuet, 1996; Parncutt, 2016). The mother's voice is probably the most salient sound (Querleu et al., 1988) because it is transmitted internally, through maternal bones and tissues, as well as externally. The fetus begins to hear at about 16–20 weeks (Hepper & Shahidullah, 1994) and becomes increasingly sensitive to the mother's voice and other patterned sounds such as melodies. At birth, infants differentiate the mother's voice from other voices, and prefer her voice to that of a stranger (DeCasper & Fifer, 1980; Hepper et al., 1993; Querleu et al., 1984). Memory for musical patterns is also evident in the late fetal period, those memories persisting, at times, after birth (Granier-Deferre et al., 2011; Hepper, 1991). These findings lend support to the role of the prenatal auditory environment in shaping newborns' responsiveness to speech and music (Fifer & Moon, 1994; Moon, 2017).

Although infants readily detect subtle changes in the pitch or duration of a single note of a musical pattern, their principal focus is on the melody and rhythm (for a review, see Trehub, 2016). Newborn infants are sensitive to the beat of rhythmic music (Winkler et al., 2009), tempo changes (Háden et al., 2015), and pitch directional changes—ascending versus descending pitch patterns (Carral et al., 2005). By 5 months of age, infants make spontaneous rhythmic movements to rhythmic music, but their movements are not synchronized with the beat (Zentner & Eerola, 2010) as they are with older listeners. Infants exhibit more movement regularity to rhythmic music played at 120 beats per minute (bpm) than at a faster tempo, suggesting a preferred tempo for infant movement (de l'Etoile et al., 2020). Passive movement to music (e.g., being bounced or rocked by others) has consequences for infants' perception of the music. When 7-month-olds are bounced on either every second or third beat of an ambiguous (i.e., unaccented) rhythm, they subsequently listen preferentially to the pattern with accents matching the experienced pattern of bouncing (Phillips-Silver & Trainor, 2005).

Infants' memory for music is particularly noteworthy. After 5-month-old infants are exposed to a vocal melody for one or two weeks but not thereafter, they recognize it 8 months later (Mehr et al., 2016). At 6 or 7 months of age, infants recognize a piano melody after hearing it at home (5 minutes daily) for a week or two, but they do not remember the original pitch level or key (Plantinga & Trainor, 2005) unless the melody is vocal (Volkova et al., 2006). The special quality of the voice and the context of exposure (e.g., home environment) make important contributions to infants' attention to music and their memory for musical details.

Like adults, infants have strong musical preferences (Cirelli & Trehub, 2018, 2020). Everyday observation reveals greater infant responsiveness to vocal compared to instrumental music, to live compared to recorded singing, and to familiar compared to unfamiliar songs. Laboratory studies reveal infants' preference for emotionally expressive renditions of songs, especially happy-sounding songs, over more neutral renditions (Corbeil et al., 2013; Trainor, 1996).

By 12 months of age, Western infants exhibit enculturation to aspects of Western rhythmic structure. Like adults, 12-month-olds perceive Western rhythms more readily than non-Western rhythms (Hannon & Trehub, 2005b), unlike 6-month-olds, who perform equally well on Western and non-Western rhythms (Hannon & Trehub, 2005a). Becoming attuned to the pitch patterns of a musical culture involves a more protracted developmental course, with sensitivity to key membership evident by 5 years of age and sensitivity to harmonic relations emerging later (Corrigall & Trainor, 2014).

In summary, the foundations of musical engagement are apparent at birth and continue to develop thereafter. Over the course of their first year, infants become increasingly captivated by music, progressively refining their skills and preferences, and acquiring some sense of culture-specific rhythmic structure. Although research to date has been conducted primarily with Western infants, the observed music processing skills are likely to be universal rather than culture specific (Mehr et al., 2019), attributable to the nature of our auditory system, the universality of music, and the ease of auditory learning.

Natural musical care: Singing to infants

As noted, *natural* musical care refers to the everyday use of music in interactions with infants. Caregivers' singing is the predominant source of *natural* musical care in infancy. Lullabies—songs for soothing infants or lulling them to sleep—are found in all known cultures (Trehub & Trainor, 1998). Western adults readily identify foreign lullabies in the context of equally slow songs from the same culture (Trehub et al., 1993). In fact, adults from a wide range of cultures are comparable in their accuracy of identifying foreign lullabies, readily distinguishing them from dance songs, healing songs, and love songs (Mehr et al., 2018). The implication is that such identification is possible because of common lullaby features across cultures. Caregivers' play songs are performed to infants at a higher pitch level, at a slower tempo, with greater temporal regularity, and with more emotive vocal tone than informal performances of the same songs in the infant's absence (Nakata & Trehub, 2011; Trainor, 1996; Trehub et al., 1997).

The expressiveness of mothers' performances for 6-month-olds depends not only on infants' presence but also on their visibility (Trehub et al., 2016); which implies that overt signs of infant engagement (e.g., wide-eyed interest) affect the emotional state of the singer and the resulting performance. Mothers smile almost constantly while singing to infants, in contrast to intermittent smiling during their speech to infants (Trehub et al., 2016). In general, mothers sing a few songs repeatedly and in a highly stereotyped manner, often with identical pitch level and tempo on different occasions (Bergeson & Trehub, 2002). The stereotypy of these performances, which enhances their memorability, makes them much like rituals in that the form of the action (e.g., ritual handwashing) may be more important than the function (e.g., cleaning hands). Rituals typically reinforce group cohesion. In a similar vein, mothers' songs function as bonding rituals, enhancing dyadic cohesion.

Although much of the research focuses on maternal singing, largely because mothers commonly serve as primary caregivers, fathers, grandparents, and others who provide regular care also sing to infants. Like mothers, fathers enhance the emotional expressiveness of their performances when singing to infants (Trehub et al., 1997). In many communities around the world, grandmothers or female elders participate actively in infant care, often serenading infants to sleep with traditional lullabies (Bezner Kerr et al., 2008; Ilari et al., 2011; Sanfilippo, 2020).

Musical experiences, regardless of geographic region or age group, are typically multimodal rather than unimodal (Savage et al., 2015). In fact, several languages designate music and dance by the same word (Bohlman, 2002). For infants who are carried throughout the day, musical experiences include simultaneous tactile sensations and movements (e.g., from maternal locomotion). Awake, alert infants in these cultures may also experience an array of visual stimuli, including the facial and limb gestures of singers.

Infants in Western urban communities have much less physical contact with mothers but much more face-to-face contact during time spent in secure devices (e.g., high chairs, bouncers, home swings) that permit hands-free caregiving. For the most part, their mothers sing lively play songs (e.g., *Itsy Bitsy Spider*, *Wheels on the Bus*), smiling almost continuously while they sing (Trehub et al., 2016), often with accompanying gestures or actions (Eckerdal & Merker, 2009). Unlike caregivers in high-contact cultures, caregivers in low-contact cultures such as North America and the United Kingdom commonly leave infants before they fall asleep, relying at times on commercial sleep machines or smartphone apps that generate white noise, nature sounds, or music to handle the challenges of infants' transition to sleep. These challenges result from infants' separation distress (i.e., separate sleeping) and their limited self-soothing repertoire (Morelli et al., 1992; Owens, 2004).

In the newborn period and thereafter, infants are more attentive to recorded singing in the maternal or infant-directed (ID) style than to informal, self-directed performances (Masataka, 1999; Trainor, 1996), the latter being less emotive. Although ID speech and singing are equally effective for *capturing* infant attention (Corbeil et al., 2013), ID singing is more effective at *sustaining* infant attention and preventing distress (Corbeil et al., 2016). Additionally, videos of ID singing are more effective than videos of ID speech for capturing and holding infant attention (Costa-Giomi, 2014; Nakata & Trehub, 2004). Not surprisingly, parents' live, multimodal performances are most effective.

If singing is effective in maintaining infants' composure, delaying the onset of distress (Corbeil et al., 2016), and modulating arousal levels (Shenfield et al., 2003) in infants who are initially calm, it may be comparably effective in soothing distressed infants. Indeed, after distress is induced in 8- and 10-month-old infants, multimodal maternal singing is more successful than multimodal maternal speech in ameliorating that distress, with familiar songs being more effective than unfamiliar songs (Cirelli & Trehub, 2020). Perhaps the familiar song and familiar performing style— the maternal bonding ritual—evoke pleasant memories of dyadic musical interactions, distracting infants from their distress.

The efficacy of maternal singing in ameliorating distress has long-term as well as short-term consequences. Caregivers' success at alleviating infant distress is predictive of infants' subsequent attachment security (Braungart-Rieker et al., 2014) and their skill in emotional self-regulation or self-soothing (Leerkes et al., 2009). Success in this regard may also increase parents' self-assurance in their caregiving role, with favourable effects on caregiver and infant well-being. Singing is also a vehicle of maternal self-care, as reflected in similar arousal-regulatory consequences of singing for mother and infant (Cirelli et al., 2019).

Maternal bonding rituals have implications beyond the mother–infant dyadic context. For example, infants as young as 5 months of age are more socially responsive to an unfamiliar woman after she sings a song from the mother's repertoire rather than a song familiarized in a non-maternal context or an unfamiliar song (Mehr et al., 2016). By 14 months of age, infants engage in a variety of prosocial behaviours: for example, offering help to others who need assistance. Some circumstances prompt them to increase their usual rate of helping. For example, 14-month-olds return more 'accidentally' dropped objects to a person who previously sang a song that their mother sometimes sang at home rather than an unfamiliar song or a rhythmic recitation of the song lyrics (Cirelli & Trehub, 2018). Perhaps infants regard those who perform a maternal ritual, however imperfectly (e.g., singing the mother's song in an atypical manner), as similar to their mother in some respects and therefore worthy of trust. These 14-month-olds also remain in closer physical proximity to the woman who sang a song than the woman who recited the song lyrics (Cirelli & Trehub, 2018). Just as singing reduces the psychological barriers between a singer and an adult audience (Pantaleoni, 1985), it may do likewise for an infant audience.

Infants also exhibit enhanced helping towards unfamiliar women whose movements are temporally aligned with their own. For example, after a woman bounces to music in or out of synchrony with 14-month-olds (who are bounced by another adult), infants offer more help to the synchronous bouncer than to the asynchronous bouncer (Cirelli et al., 2014). In this case, the synchronous mover may seem more attuned to them and, consequently, a superior social partner. The consequences of interpersonal synchrony for prosocial behaviour are evident beyond infancy (see examples in the Musical care in childhood chapter).

Infants' engagement with singing extends beyond active music listening. Rudimentary singing often begins within months of infants' first birthday, initially involving periodic vocalizations coupled with iconic actions (e.g., finger movements during *Itsy Bitsy Spider*) during maternal performances. Mothers often initiate singing games in which they omit the last word of each line (e.g., *Twinkle, Twinkle, Little _____*), prompting infants to supply the missing sounds (Trehub & Gudmundsdottir, 2019). Infants fill the gap with word-like vocalizations that incorporate accurate timing but inaccurate pitch. Independent singing commonly occurs by their second birthday, at which time infants sing their caregiver's typical songs. At that point, their relatively accurate reproduction of pitch contours and timing results in recognizable tunes (Gudmundsdottir & Trehub, 2018).

Independent singing is much more than a musical milestone. It is also an emotional milestone, providing infants with an important tool for emotional self-regulation. By singing the mother's songs in her absence, infants can reinstate some of the pleasant feelings linked to those bonding rituals, thereby decreasing the stress of separation. Many toddlers sing in the solitude of their crib, capitalizing on opportunities for self-soothing, musical practice, and improvisation (Sole, 2017).

In summary, *natural* musical care, and singing in particular, serves a variety of functions for infants and their caregivers. It regulates arousal levels in both partners (Cirelli et al., 2019), ameliorates infant distress (Cirelli & Trehub, 2020), enhances dyadic bonds (Trehub & Russo, 2020), and promotes healthy social and emotional development (Cirelli & Trehub, 2018). It achieves these objectives, in part, by the inherent repetition and temporal predictability of music (Margulis, 2014), by caregivers' highly stereotyped and emotive performances (Bergeson & Trehub, 2002; Trehub et al., 2016), by their use of highly familiar musical materials (Cirelli & Trehub, 2020), and their multimodal performances being attuned to cultural norms and infants' momentary needs (Trehub & Russo, 2020). When circumstances preclude live, multimodal performances, solitary music listening manages to provide comfort and solace to infants and adults, functioning much like a social surrogate (Corbeil et al., 2016; Schäfer et al., 2020). The nature and consequences of such natural musical engagement have implications for the use of music in targeted or therapeutic contexts.

Targeted musical care: Interventions and music therapy

During pregnancy, *targeted* musical care aims to enhance maternal and fetal well-being, with potential carryover effects in the postnatal period. Postnatally, *targeted* musical care supports caregivers' needs, infants' needs, and the caregiver–infant relationship. Finally, musical care with vulnerable infants targets those with disabilities and prematurely born infants in the neonatal intensive care unit (NICU).

Targeted musical care for maternal health

Musical interventions have been used to support maternal physical health. For example, music listening in pregnancy reduces elevated maternal blood pressure (Cao et al., 2016; Meenakshi, 2016), with elevated levels having potentially dangerous consequences for the mother and her infant. Music listening and music therapy also reduce pain, stress, and anxiety during childbirth and caesarean section (for a review see Wulff et al., 2017). Additionally, songs and storytelling have been used productively for the dissemination of information about maternal and infant health, especially in low- and middle-income countries where maternal and infant health problems present ongoing challenges (World Health Organization, 2015). According to Silver (2001), such approaches succeed because of the engaging context, the credibility of information embedded within local practices, and the simple, easily learned songs, all of which add to the sustainability of the messaging. Group music making—participatory dancing and singing—involving community women's groups (Prost et al., 2013) can help merge traditional and medical models to enhance maternal and infant physical health. This type of hybrid health communication has been documented in several countries (e.g., Bingley, 2011; Quadros & Dorstewitz, 2011; Silver, 2001).

One example of this hybrid model involves the Kanyeleng women in The Gambia. Traditional Kanyeleng groups consist of women who have experienced infertility or child mortality (McConnell, 2015, 2020). Kanyeleng groups participate in prayer, disguise, trickery, music performance, and rituals aimed at preventing infertility and infant mortality (McConnell, 2020; Skramstad, 2008). Although many Kanyeleng groups continue to practice traditional beliefs and rituals, they have begun to as-sume prominent roles as health communicators, supported by the Ministry of Health (McConnell, 2020). Kanyeleng groups perform in and beyond their local commu-nities, disseminating information about HIV/AIDS (McConnell, 2015), vaccina-tions (McConnell, 2017), diarrhoea, female genital cutting (FGC), and breastfeeding (McConnell, 2016), all of which are relevant for pregnant women and new mothers. The Kanyeleng groups' historical and continuing focus on women's reproductive health, coupled with their expertise as musicians and health communicators, pro-vides a potent example of traditional musical rituals used in conjunction with con-temporary medical knowledge to foster enhanced maternal and infant health. The Kanyeleng experience may be instructive for public health authorities in Western countries, who are often unsuccessful in communicating health messages to mi-nority, marginalized, or seldom-heard groups in their midst.

Music interventions can also support maternal mental health during pregnancy and after birth in a non-stigmatizing, accessible, and cost-effective manner. For women with low-risk pregnancies (i.e., no diagnosed mental or physical challenges), a two-week music listening intervention lowers self-reported levels of stress relative to no intervention (Chang et al., 2015). Similarly, a two-week music therapy inter-vention during pregnancy reduces stress, anxiety, and depressive symptoms rela-tive to a no-treatment control group (Chang et al., 2008). Even solitary listening to relaxing music is more effective than silent relaxation for decreasing anxiety in preg-nant women (Nwebube et al., 2017). A recent study in The Gambia investigated the effects of music groups on anxiety and depression in a community sample of pregnant women (Sanfilippo, 2020). The aforementioned Kanyeleng groups co-developed and led participatory music sessions with a group of pregnant women from their com-munity, an intervention that was acceptable to facilitators and participants. The ses-sions, which involved all of the participants singing and dancing together, included songs created by the Kanyeleng groups that communicated important information about ways to seek help, lifted the women's mood, and created a socially supportive network (Sanfilippo et al., 2020). Women who participated in the music group in addition to standard care—four or more visits with a midwife—showed reduced symptoms of anxiety and depression relative to participants who received standard care only (Sanfilippo et al., 2020). Additionally, in a recent three-armed randomized control trial, researchers investigated the effects of listening to relaxing music, versus participation in a singing class led by a music therapist, compared with treatment as usual on maternal well-being and mother–infant bonding (Wulff et al., 2021). The researchers found that both the singing and listening intervention showed positive effects on stress, with a greater reduction of cortisol levels and an increase in oxytocin. They also found that the singing group showed a larger reduction in cortisol com-pared to the music listening group and a greater increase in general self-efficacy and perceived closeness to the unborn child. However, they found no significant effects on depressive symptoms, potentially because of low levels of symptoms at baseline in their sample. Although these intervention studies indicate the potential of musical care for managing stress and anxiety during pregnancy across diverse contexts, there is little research in this domain. In view of the limited options for addressing potentially problematic levels of stress, anxiety, and depression in pregnancy, further research in this area is warranted.

High levels of prenatal anxiety and depression affect roughly 10–20% of women, which is comparable to the incidence of postpartum depression (Milgrom et al., 2008). Moreover, maternal mental health problems can have adverse effects on fetal and infant development (Glover, 2015). Because prenatal anxiety and depression are the best predictors of postpartum depression (Milgrom et al., 2008; Robertson et al., 2004), interventions that target symptomatic pregnant women may support women during pregnancy and influence postnatal outcomes for mother and child. High stress levels during pregnancy also affect fetal and infant development (Braithwaite et al., 2015; Glover et al., 2010), in part, by altering the uterine environment (Bergman et al., 2010). For example, maternal anxiety is thought to increase the transfer of maternal cortisol (a hormonal index of stress) to the fetus (Glover, 2015). Cortisol levels in amniotic fluid are inversely correlated with infant cognitive development (Bergman et al., 2010), with high stress levels during pregnancy increasing the risk of cognitive and behavioural problems in infancy (Glover et al., 2009). Additionally, maternal stress and depression can have adverse effects on infant attachment security (Coyl et al., 2002), with implications for infant developmental outcomes (Murray et al., 1996). In principle, musical care for pregnant women, even those with low-risk pregnancies, could foster positive mood, influencing subsequent outcomes for mother and infant. To date, however, there is no evidence that prenatal musical care enhances maternal attachment to the fetus (Chang et al., 2015; Persico et al., 2017; Shin & Kim, 2011). Nevertheless, interventions involving directed music listening or music therapy in low-risk pregnancies show promise in promoting well-being during pregnancy. Although such interventions may be beneficial, it is prudent to allocate resources where they are most needed—pregnant women experiencing moderately elevated to high levels of anxiety and depression.

In the postpartum period, musical engagement is effective in ameliorating maternal depression and anxiety (Fancourt & Perkins, 2018; Terry & Terry, 2012). A recent randomized control trial revealed that a 10-week singing group for women with postpartum depression resulted in greater reduction in depressive symptoms than a non-singing playgroup (Fancourt & Perkins, 2018). These singing groups provide mothers with a creative experience, skills for calming babies, immersive 'me time', a sense of achievement and identity, and enhanced bonding with their infants (Perkins et al., 2018).

As noted, lullabies and other ID songs provide an important channel for meaningful and sensitive interactions between mother and infant, comforting each partner (Cirelli et al., 2019; Friedman et al., 2010) and enriching mother–infant bonds (Milligan et al., 2003). Postpartum depression impedes dyadic interaction, putting infants at risk of dysregulation. Depressed mothers often exhibit less sensitive and less timely responses to infant signals, resulting in lesser affective attunement to infants than non-depressed mothers (Donovan et al., 1998; Goodman et al., 1993; Marwick & Murray, 2009). Their infants may exhibit elevated physiological arousal as well as diminished attention and cognitive processing (Beeghly et al., 2016; Pound, 2005). A depressed interaction style on the part of infants complicates dyadic interactions by creating a dynamic of reciprocal deficiencies in reading and responding to social and emotional cues (Beeghly et al., 2016; Speranza et al., 2006).

Depressed mothers can benefit from interventions designed to enhance their sensitivity to infant affect and arousal (Bargiel, 2004). Mothers with postpartum depression tend to sing faster to infants than mothers without depression (de l'Etoile & Leider, 2011), failing to exhibit the characteristic tempo slowing of typical maternal singing (Trainor, 1996; Trehub et al., 1997). In general, their performances are less emotionally expressive than those of non-depressed mothers, less affectively attuned to infants, and somewhat robotic.

Like other infants, however, infants of depressed mothers exhibit sustained gaze at their mother (de l'Etoile, 2012) or at a stranger (music therapist) who sings the same song as the mother, indicating the efficacy of ID singing in maintaining infant engagement regardless of singer familiarity. In short, ID singing enhances mother–infant interaction even in the context of postpartum depression. The responsiveness of infants of depressed mothers to the ID singing of a music therapist supports the concept of interventions based on interaction coaching (de l'Etoile, 2006b; O'Gorman, 2007). For example, a music therapist can model ID singing for the depressed mother by singing in a manner that reflects the infant's state or modifies the infant's state (de l'Etoile, 2012). Through guided therapeutic discussion, the mother learns to identify infant responses to musical elements in the therapist's singing. The therapist subsequently provides sensitive encouragement, guidance, and support for maternal singing to infants.

Van Puyvelde et al. (2014) conducted a five-week musical intervention (weekly sessions) for four mother–infant dyads in an inpatient setting for the treatment of severe postpartum depression. The program, led by two performing artists, used components of music, singing, and movement to promote mother–infant intersubjectivity or shared engagement. Participating dyads increased their frequency and duration of mutual engagement from the first to the fifth and final session.

Targeted musical care shows considerable promise for reducing emotional distress, prenatally and postnatally, and enhancing mother–infant interaction. For mothers experiencing distress during pregnancy and after birth, musical care provides a valuable supplement to more conventional forms of physical and mental health care.

Targeted musical care for infants

During the last trimester of pregnancy, music is audible to the fetus, affecting fetal movement (Kafali et al., 2011), heart rate (Oh et al., 2016), and respiration (Zimmer et al., 1982). Though a variety of commercial music devices (e.g., pregnancy music belts) target parents during pregnancy, research has shown that these devices are not helpful in supporting the complex multimodal maturation of the fetal sensory system (Jahn et al., 2016). Additionally, research on the use of music devices in pregnancy and after birth has highlighted the importance of ensuring that the sound levels of these devices do not pose risks for fetal and infant hearing (Graven & Browne, 2008; Hugh et al., 2014). Therefore, traditional implementation of music listening and maternal singing appear preferable to the use of such devices.

Although evidence is limited, research on prenatal *targeted* musical care has shown some benefits for infant health and development. For example, music listening for 1 hour daily during pregnancy predicted better newborn orientation skills, state regulation, and autonomic stability (Arya et al., 2012). In another study, 167 pregnant women at 24 weeks of gestation were assigned to a prenatal group that encouraged lullaby singing prenatally and postnatally or a control group featuring comparable classes but no mention of singing (Persico et al., 2017). In the first month after birth, mothers in the lullaby group sang more and their infants cried less than those in the control group, as indicated by maternal self-report. In addition, mothers reported experiencing less stress and stronger bonds with their infants. To better understand the potential impact of prenatal musical care for fetal and infant development, more longitudinal research is necessary.

Targeted musical care after birth addresses the needs of the developing infant by focusing on the mother–infant relationship. In this regard, musical care aims to promote infants' self-regulation of mood and arousal level (Beeghly et al., 2016; Beer & Lombardo, 2009; Vohs & Baumeister, 2004). Because of their limited self-regulatory skills, young infants rely on caregivers to respond to their signals, thereby experiencing 'co-regulation' or 'mutual regulation' (Beeghly et al., 2016; Feldman, 2007; Sroufe, 2000). Effective dyadic interactions can lead infants to integrate caregivers' successful responses into their own repertoire, facilitating infants' transition to emotional self-regulation (Calkin & Hill, 2007). Infants who experience sensitive and responsive caregiving become more effective at managing situational stress and modulating their own arousal levels (Beeghly et al., 2016; Calkin & Hill, 2007).

Sensitive caregiving enables infants to experience affective attunement, which involves the coordination of parent–infant gaze, affective displays, vocalizations, and body movement (Berger, 2011). This attunement can be experienced through simultaneous or sequential dyadic behaviours, as when caregiver and infant respond to each other in a chain of matching or related behaviours. These coordinated interactions resemble a well-timed 'dance' between the partners as they move towards desirable levels of affective engagement. For infants, such well-timed exchanges promote positive arousal, which fuels the development of self-regulation (Feldman, 2007). These coordinated interactions are fundamentally temporal, unfolding systematically over time. Time or temporality, a central parameter of effective communication and emotion regulation, is a defining feature of music. In that sense, parent–infant interactions are often considered musical, a phenomenon known as 'communicative musicality' (Malloch, 1999; Malloch & Trevarthen, 2009) a concept that will be used throughout the life stages in following chapters. In dyads that do not readily achieve affective attunement, well-designed musical experiences, with their intrinsically temporal and expressive nature, can guide parents towards sensitive caregiving that promotes infant self-regulation (Edwards, 2011; Wheeler & Stultz, 2008).

Disruptions of caregiver–infant interaction increase infants' risk for inadequate self-regulation (Beeghly et al., 2016; Edwards, 2011; Van Puyvelde et al., 2014). Prematurely born infants, for example, are often unable to respond to maternal behaviours, whereas infants with disabilities can be delayed in their ability to engage with caregivers. As noted, mothers with postpartum depression may struggle, temporarily or chronically, to successfully contribute to co-regulation (Bargiel, 2004). In these instances, music therapy interventions can enhance caregivers' sensitivity to infant affect and arousal, promoting positive interactions. Ideally, the design and application of such interventions should be guided by theory and empirical evidence.

To experience co-regulation, infants must direct their attention and modulate their arousal levels (Berger, 2011; Gross & Thompson, 2007; Thompson, 1994), implicating neural structures that exert top-down and bottom-up influences (Beeghly et al., 2016). Self-regulation and music listening share a common network of neural structures involved in the deployment of attention and the processing of emotional stimuli. (Banfield et al., 2004; Calkin & Hill, 2007; Payne & Bachevalier, 2009). These neural structures, which are also critical for emotional responses to music (Blood & Zatorre, 2001; Menon & Levitin, 2005), develop throughout infancy, a process mediated by caregiver interaction (Schore, 2000). Experience with music is thought to 'exercise' the brain areas implicated in self-regulation. As noted, mothers around the world provide *natural* musical care in the form of singing to infants, doing so in a way that captures infants' attention, reflects or modifies their state or arousal level (de l'Etoile, 2006a; Nakata & Trehub, 2011), and promotes co-regulation and bonding.

Although responses to ID singing are well documented for TD infants, that is not the case for infants with special needs whose self-regulation and co-regulation skills may be compromised. The ability of ID singing to maintain composure (Corbeil et al., 2016) and reduce distress in TD infants (Cirelli & Trehub, 2020) provides encouragement for its use with at-risk infants and caregivers. Achieving positive outcomes with at-risk populations depends on caregivers' ability to recognize signs of infant overstimulation or discomfort (e.g., grimacing, eye clenching, eye rubbing, gaze aversion, back arching) and to adjust their singing accordingly (de l'Etoile, 2008; Standley, 1991; Standley & Whipple, 2003). In effect, *natural* musical care, especially ID singing, provides the theoretical foundation for the development of music interventions and music therapy for at-risk infants. In the following sections, we summarize research, primarily from music therapy and music psychology, indicating how *targeted* musical care benefits special populations, such as infants with disabilities and premature infants.

Musical care and Down syndrome

Infants with cerebral palsy, autism spectrum disorder, Down syndrome (DS), developmental delays, or other disabilities commonly have difficulty experiencing mutual regulation (Wheeler & Stultz, 2008). Their caregivers are vulnerable to social isolation and parenting stress, which can adversely affect parenting, compounding infants' risk for dysregulation (Williams et al., 2012). Infants with DS have reduced volume in cortical and subcortical structures linked to attention and arousal (relative to TD infants), increasing the challenges of self-regulation (Jernigan et al., 1993; Pinter et al., 2001). As a result, they may seem passive or disinterested in interactions with caregivers, leading caregivers, at times, to adopt an interaction style of 'forceful warmth' (Carvajal & Iglesias, 2006; Moore et al., 2008; Slonims & McConachie, 2006). By doing so, caregivers may miss important infant cues and fail to optimize infant arousal, jeopardizing the development of infant self-regulation (Spiker, 2006).

Nevertheless, caregivers' ID singing to infants with DS appears to be sensitive to their distinct attentional and arousal needs. In comparison with mothers of TD infants, mothers of DS infants sing at a higher maximum pitch and use more key changes during play songs, perhaps to garner infants' attention or optimize their arousal (de l'Etoile et al., 2017). They also take longer to establish a steady pulse in their lullabies and play songs than do mothers of TD infants. Because infants with DS are often slow to respond during caregiving interactions (Carvajal & Iglesias, 2006; Cicchetti et al., 1991), mothers may take longer to interpret infant behaviour before establishing rhythmic song structure. Nevertheless, their performances are high in emotional expressiveness, like those of other mothers, so they are likely to support affect regulation. Indeed, maternal singing to DS and TD infants elicits sustained gaze at their mother, confirming its efficacy in maintaining their attention (de l'Etoile, 2015). In fact, infants with DS sustain their gaze somewhat longer than TD peers and display less intermittent gaze—alternating their focus between mother and objects in the environment—than their TD counterparts. Infants with DS and TD peers display neutral affect during ID singing, which is characteristic of young infants during face-to-face interaction with caregivers (Van Puyvelde et al., 2013). Neutral affect in these instances may reflect interest or relaxation coupled with moderate arousal levels and moderately positive valence.

Overall, these exploratory studies provide insight into mothers' and infants' ID singing that can inform future interventions. Caregivers of infants with DS should be encouraged to sing as a means of focusing infants' attention and regulating their arousal levels. A music therapist could provide guidance about the unique musical needs of infants with DS and manage parents' expectations regarding infant responsiveness.

Musical care and other special needs

Music therapists have used short-term group interventions to help support caregivers and their infants with disabilities or special needs. Sing & Grow, a well-known Australian music program, is designed for caregivers and young children (0 to 5 years) with social disadvantages, very young parents, or parents of children with a disability (Nicholson et al., 2008; Williams et al., 2012). The program, which is implemented by music therapists, uses music-based play activities to promote child development. It encourages parental responsiveness and the use of developmentally appropriate parenting skills. Positive outcomes of the program include reductions in parents' mental health symptoms and increases in children's communication and social skills. Specifically, caregivers who complete the program exhibit greater acceptance of their situation, greater sensitivity to their child, and more effective parent–child engagement.

Walworth (2009) devised a developmentally appropriate music therapy program for caregivers and their prematurely born infants or full-term infants with disabilities (e.g., visual impairment, developmental delay). The program, which uses live music, provides opportunities for children to meet developmental milestones through social learning in a group setting: for example, by observing actions and behaviours modelled by parents and music therapists (Pineda et al., 2017). Future work could explore the impact of musical care on stress and anxiety reduction in parents of infants with special needs or vulnerabilities.

Musical care in the Neonatal Intensive Care Unit (NICU)

Infants born prematurely or at term with high-risk conditions receive life-saving interventions in a NICU. This environment presents unique challenges, both acoustically—intense, unpredictable sounds—and otherwise—frequent invasive procedures over the course of weeks or months (Anderson & Patel, 2018; Cruz et al., 2016; Ettenberger, 2017). Premature infants lack the regulatory mechanisms for coping with this chaotic environment, and their hospitalization precludes unlimited access to parents or caregivers (Anderson & Patel, 2018; Shoemark et al., 2015). In short, these infants experience ongoing stress at a vulnerable developmental period, heightening their risk for short- and long-term dysregulation.

According to Anderson and Patel (2018), music can ameliorate some of the adverse effects of the NICU by reducing stress; providing a surrogate, supportive social signal (e.g., maternal or ID singing); and providing environmental enrichment. The repeated presentation of lullabies, with their predictable structure, simplicity, steady rhythms, descending melodic contours, and familiarity, may help infants organize their responses, potentially modulating arousal and affect for more effective physiological regulation (Olischar et al., 2011; Shoemark et al., 2015; Ullsten et al., 2016).

This theoretical foundation of musical care in the NICU informs the development of therapeutic interventions for premature and high-risk infants. Gooding (2010) identifies musical experiences considered appropriate and beneficial for neonates, according to specific developmental stages.

1. *Survival/pacification stage.* During this stage, which lasts until the infant reaches ~2.5 lbs (1.13 kg) and demonstrates signs of adequate neurological development, no-contact music listening is advisable: for example, recorded lullabies

and/or the mother's voice presented at a modest volume (below 70 dB). The goal is to improve physiological markers such as stable oxygen saturation levels (Cevasco & Grant, 2005).

2. *Cautious stimulation phase.* During this stage, which spans approximately 30 to 32 weeks' gestational age, the use of music, alone or in conjunction with kangaroo care (i.e., skin-to-skin contact) or multimodal stimulation (MMS: music combined with stroking, rocking, and eye contact), can soothe infants and increase their tolerance of stimulation. MMS reportedly leads to earlier NICU discharge (Standley, 1998) and improved parent–infant interaction (Whipple, 2000).

3. *Interactive learning phase.* At roughly 32 weeks' gestational age, music can be used in the context of inconsolable crying, procedural pain, and feeding. Inconsolable crying, which may result from inadequate self-regulation, expends valuable energy (i.e., burning calories needed for weight gain), potentially interfering with neurological development and increasing parental stress, with negative consequences for the parent–infant relationship.

Recorded singing—unaccompanied lullabies with simple rhythms, melodies, and harmonies and soft timbre—seems to reduce inconsolable crying and improve heart rate, respiration rate, and oxygen saturation in premature infants (Keith et al., 2009). The authors suggest that live music may be even more effective because of the possibility of contingent responding to infant behaviour, but their results support the use of recorded music when a music therapist or caregiver is unavailable.

Recorded music has also been used to address procedural pain in the NICU (Cavaiuolo et al., 2015). Infants who hear classical instrumental (violin) music with major tonality, consonance, a single melodic line, and slow tempo (50–60 bpm) exhibit reductions in heart rate and distress as well as increased oxygen saturation levels.

Premature infants must exhibit adequate oral feeding skills before discharge from the NICU (Chorna et al., 2014). To that end, non-nutritive sucking enhances oral feeding and can be developed through practice and behavioural conditioning: for example, by contingent presentation of recorded music (Gooding, 2010). Chorna et al. (2014) used a pacifier-activated music player that enabled premature infants to hear recordings of their mothers singing lullabies, contingent upon non-nutritive sucking, prior to scheduled feeding times. Infants showed improvements in oral feeding rate, volume of oral intake, and number of oral feedings per day as well as increased sucking pressure relative to a control group receiving standard care.

Ullsten and colleagues (Ullsten et al., 2017) examined the effect of live lullaby singing on the physiological and affective responses of premature infants in the NICU during venipuncture (i.e., heel prick). The lullabies, parent-preferred or traditional versions in parents' native language, were sung by a music therapy student. Microanalysis of infant behaviour before, during, and after the procedure revealed more stable and more regular responses to live singing in combination with standard care compared to standard care only.

4. *Infant stimulation phase.* In this final developmental stage, Gooding (2010) recommends increasing physical contact with infants (e.g., cuddling) and the use of stimulating music to promote non-cry vocalizations, eye contact, and communication.

In general, musical exposure in the NICU is considered safe and relevant for promoting positive infant outcomes (Pineda et al., 2017), especially in regard to pacification and stabilization, as indicated by physiological and behavioural measures (Haslbeck, 2012a; O'Toole et al., 2017; Palazzi et al., 2018; van der Heijden et al., 2016). Nevertheless, the utility of music in the NICU remains controversial. Although music therapy in the NICU has been explored across a range of cultures and geographic areas (for a review, see Shoemark & Ettenberger, 2020), often with favourable consequences, a meta-analysis of rigorously designed studies (randomized controlled trials of music therapy compared with standard care, alternative interventions, or placebo) found robust effects on infant respiration and maternal anxiety but no other behavioural or physiological effects (Bieleninik et al., 2016). Confirmation of other reported benefits of music therapy in the NICU is impeded by the paucity of systematic clinical trials in this domain. Until such trials, which build on protocols such as those discussed in the next section, are available and reveal consistent benefits, the use of music therapy in this setting will remain limited.

Music therapy protocol in the NICU

Recorded music may help preterm or high-risk infants maintain homeostasis, but it lacks the contingent responding of a sensitive caregiver (Malloch et al., 2012). When recorded music is used, however, earphones or other similar devices may be precluded because of possible adverse effects (Graven, 2000). Live music, by contrast, offers greater potential benefit because of its sensitivity to infants' momentary needs and greater scope for stress reduction (Garunkstiene et al., 2014; Palazzi et al., 2018; van der Heijden et al., 2016). Live musical interventions often involve lullaby singing by a caregiver or music therapist, with or without instrumental accompaniment, and several measures of infant physiological and behavioural outcome (Heitmann et al., 2016; Schlez et al., 2011). In a landmark study involving a randomized multisite trial, live singing of parent-preferred lullabies sustained quiet-alert states in NICU infants, and live playing of a Gato box (slit drum that emits soothing tones) reduced infant heart rate and increased sucking and feeding behaviours (Loewy et al., 2013). NICU music interventions are best coordinated by music therapists who can intervene directly with the infant, the mother–infant dyad, and other family members (Anderson & Patel, 2018; Haslbeck, 2012a; Palazzi et al., 2018).

Following careful assessment of infant needs, music therapists can provide music interventions that are safe and appropriate, increasing the likelihood of positive therapeutic outcomes (Bargiel, 2004). In *natural* musical care, mothers intuitively adjust their singing to match or alter infant state. With *targeted* musical care for premature or high-risk infants, the music therapist modifies the musical features to accommodate infants' needs and capacity for responding. Such 'contingent singing' or control of musical elements provides interaction that is attuned to infant and family needs, avoiding overstimulation and reflecting the family's cultural, ethnic, or religious beliefs (Anderson & Patel, 2018; Haslbeck, 2012a; Shoemark & Grocke, 2010).

In view of the stresses facing parents after the birth of a premature or high-risk infant, interventions for infants should involve the family whenever possible (Ettenberger, 2017; Palazzi et al., 2018). A music therapist can help parents gain confidence in handling and caring for their infant as well as reading and responding to the infant's cues (Malloch et al., 2012; Shoemark & Dearn, 2008). A number of experts recommend training parents in the NICU to provide contingent musical interactions that have been shown to accommodate and stabilize infants' vital signs in the hospital setting and at home (Ettenberger, 2017; Loewy, 2015). Parental singing in the NICU is also self-soothing, lessening parents' feelings of fear, anxiety, or grief (Loewy, 2015). Furthermore, infants' responsiveness to such singing provides critical validation of their parental role (McLean et al., 2019).

Evidence for family-centred musical care in the NICU is limited but promising. Following participation in highly structured parent–infant music sessions, infant NICU graduates exhibit improved cognition, communication, and motor skills, compared with no-treatment controls (Hamm et al., 2017). The music sessions include developmental coaching and guided parental activities that scaffold infant progress and support parent–infant interaction. To determine the long-term impact of NICU music therapy, Ghetti et al. (2019) launched LongSTEP (a longitudinal study of music therapy's effectiveness for premature infants and their caregivers), an international, randomized clinical trial with a family-centred approach that emphasizes parental singing to accommodate infant state, promote parent–infant co-regulation, and bonding. Over a 24-month period, LongSTEP researchers conduct periodic assessments of infants' cognitive, communication, motor, and social/emotional development, as well as maternal depression, parental anxiety, and stress. This LongSTEP approach includes observation and dialogue on infant and parent needs, the use of voice, especially parental voice, as the main musical source, the encouragement of active parental participation, the modification of music in response to infant states and cues, and the integration of the family's culture and music preferences (Gaden et al., 2021). It is designed to support infants and parents in the NICU and beyond, as they transition to home and community, and has already been shown to be feasible across two European countries (Bieleninik et al., 2020; Ghetti et al., 2021).

Unquestionably, music therapy interventions in the NICU would benefit from more rigorous and focused research. To optimize favourable outcomes, such as infant and dyadic regulation, and to minimize infant overstimulation, future research should be based on premature/high-risk infants' physiologic and sensory needs as well as therapeutic mechanisms underlying the efficacy of music (Graven, 2000). From this foundation, researchers should identify the most beneficial and sustainable outcomes for infants, including short- and long-term neurodevelopmental effects (Anderson & Patel, 2018; Bieleninik et al., 2016; Haslbeck, 2012a). Moreover, research protocols should be consistent in terms of type and duration of intervention, therapeutic providers, and patient demographics (Chorna et al., 2014; a). When possible, design and measurement should incorporate mixed methods to capture the complexities of parent and infant behaviour (Haslbeck, 2012a), with considerations of clinical as well as statistical significance to ensure the practical relevance of such interventions (Palazzi et al., 2018). In the interest of developing the most effective interventions, research protocols should be further informed by input from interdisciplinary teams that include neonatologists, music therapists, nursing staff, and family representatives (Pineda et al., 2017).

Our current understanding of *natural* and *targeted* musical care reflects the efforts of multiple disciplines, including ethnomusicology, music therapy, music psychology, developmental psychology, psychiatry, obstetrics, and paediatrics, involving different facets of music in the care of infants and caregivers. Research and practice in this domain show promise as a broadly applicable and cost-effective model of care from pregnancy through infancy. Admittedly, there are significant gaps in knowledge that include cultural components of musical care and optimal means of delivery in therapeutic settings.

A call for interdisciplinary collaboration

This chapter presents work from a range of scholarly and clinical disciplines that share an interest in understanding and promoting musical care in infancy, including therapeutic applications of music. Various disciplines have made important contributions, but greater progress could be achieved by collaborative or interdisciplinary efforts, with considerate benefit for infants, caregivers, families, and communities.

Women's standard care during pregnancy and after birth currently involves input from a variety of experts in maternal health, perinatal mental health, and paediatrics, but greater collaboration between scholars and clinicians is desirable. Moreover, parent involvement is critical (Barham, 2011). Because musical care in infancy occurs within a cultural and social context, researchers and clinicians should design and implement interventions that are sensitive to parents' caregiving and musical preferences. Such interventions are likely to be most successful when parents are recognized as collaborative partners striving towards common goals. However, the challenges of interdisciplinary and patient cooperation are considerable, including differences in priorities and terminology, resource limitations, and time (Haslbeck, 2012b; Lillas & Turnbull, 2009; Schetter & Glynn, 2010).

Future directions

The findings from studies of *natural* and *targeted* musical care provide inspiration for future investigations and applications of musical care in infancy. With respect to *natural* musical care, we know much more about Western practices than about non-Western practices. Although there has been little study of infant musical care in non-Western contexts, information about other aspects of infant care from these contexts can inform *natural* as well as *targeted* musical care in Western contexts. In agrarian societies, for example, mothers tend to hold or carry infants almost constantly (LeVine, 1988), one consequence of which is reduced crying relative to Western infants (Hunziker & Barr, 1986). Moreover, ID vocalizations in such contexts, whether spoken or sung, tend to be soothing (Trehub & Prince, 2010) and accompanied by physical contact, unlike the usual arousing ID songs of Western mothers, which commonly occur in face-to-face contexts (see Trehub & Russo, 2020). Some of these differences stem from cultural values about interdependence, as opposed to independence (Rothbaum et al., 2000).

As noted, lessons from the use of musical care in health communication may be applicable to immigrant or minority communities in Western nations so that important information about pregnancy, infant care, and self-care can be disseminated by trusted sources in a respectful manner. Moreover, the mood-enhancing and anxiety-reducing effects of music justify continued research related to maternal and infant mental health. In view of the high incidence of prenatal and postpartum depression and anxiety and their impact on infant development, further research could pave the way for evidence-based interventions. Regarding infants with disabilities, musical care in infancy can help parents recognize and respond to their infant's unique cues and needs. Here again, evidence-based protocols are necessary to ensure optimal delivery of care that reduces parental distress and supports parent–infant engagement.

With respect to music therapy in the NICU, the diversity of standards and practices impedes greater adoption of such interventions. In view of the complexities of music therapy in NICU care, experts emphasize the necessity of interdisciplinary collaboration among medical personnel, music therapists, and families. Only when collaborative NICU research by physicians and music therapists appears in medical journals is music therapy likely to become part of standard care in the NICU.

For the most part, research on infant musical care has focused mainly on the mother as the agent of care. This emphasis may not result from selection bias on the part of researchers but rather from self-selection by non-clinical volunteers for research. In fact, fathers' singing to infants is as emotionally expressive as that of mothers even though fathers sing less frequently to infants (Trehub et al., 1997). For clinical populations such as premature infants, high-risk infants, and infants with disabilities, it is desirable to include those who provide (or will provide) regular or intermittent care for infants (e.g., fathers, partners, grandparents), for the benefit of all. Family-centred care in the NICU (Gooding et al., 2011) is therefore a suitable model for *targeted* musical care.

Among the challenges of health and musical care for parents and infants are barriers to access, especially for families from marginalized or seldom-heard communities. Impediments to access result in staggering disparities between advantaged and disadvantaged groups in infant and maternal outcomes (Kogan et al., 1994; Lu &

Halfon, 2003; Pickett et al., 2009). Culturally embedded and community-based interventions increase the accessibility, sustainability, and impact of such interventions (Lassi & Bhutta, 2015; Rahman et al., 2013). Future research and practice in musical care during infancy could use existing community music groups and organizations to deliver interventions aimed at supporting infants and caregivers in marginalized or seldom-heard communities.

Conclusion

This chapter highlighted the relevance of musical care for infants and their caregivers. Infants are motivated music listeners who engage with and learn from music in their daily lives. Musical caregiving rituals, involving singing to infants, occur in every known culture and have beneficial consequences for infant and caregiver. Beyond such *natural* musical care, *targeted* musical care, involving music interventions and music therapy, can support infants and caregivers in the context of various challenges. In vulnerable communities that have limited trust of the formal medical system or levels of low literacy, musical care can provide a culturally sensitive channel for disseminating information about physical and mental health. *Targeted* musical care can also confer benefits on mothers with anxiety and depression, infants with disabilities, infants in the NICU and their parents. Further research, ideally interdisciplinary and family-centred, is necessary to ascertain optimal modes of intervention and to develop standardized, evidence-based protocols for use with special or vulnerable populations. In addition, cross-cultural examples of *natural* musical care can provide insights into the delivery of *targeted* musical care. Finally, it is important to remove barriers—financial, cultural, and social—to the accessibility of musical care.

References

Anderson, D. E., & Patel, A. D. (2018). Infants born preterm, stress, and neurodevelopment in the neonatal intensive care unit: Might music have an impact? *Developmental Medicine and Child Neurology, 60*(3), 256–266. https://doi.org/10.1111/dmcn.13663

Arya, R., Chansoria, M., Konanki, R., & Tiwari, D. K. (2012). Maternal music exposure during pregnancy influences neonatal behaviour: An open-label randomized controlled trial. *International Journal of Pediatrics, 901812*, 1–6. https://doi.org/10.1155/2012/901812

Banfield, J. F., Wyland, C. L., Macrae, C. N., Munte, T. F., & Heatherton, T. F. (2004). The cognitive neuroscience of self-regulation. In Kathleen D. Vohs & R. F. Baumeister (Eds.), *Handbook of self-regulation: Research, theory, and applications* (pp. 62–83). Guilford Press. https://doi.org/10.1136/jnnp.2003.018713

Bargiel, M. (2004). Lullabies and play songs: Theoretical considerations for an early attachment music therapy intervention through parental singing for developmentally at-risk infants. *Voices: A World Forum for Music Therapy, 4*(1). https://doi.org/10.15845/voices.v4i1.149

Barham, L. (2011). Public and patient involvement at the UK National Institute for Health and Clinical Excellence. *The Patient: Patient-Centred Outcomes Research, 4*(1), 1–10. https://doi.org/10.2165/11586090-000000000-00000

Beeghly, M., Perry, B. D., & Tronick, E. Z. (2016). Self-regulatory processes in early development. In S. Maltzman (Ed.), *The Oxford handbook of treatment processes and outcomes in psychology: A multidisciplinary, biopsychosocial approach* (pp. 42–54). Oxford University Press. https://doi.org/10.1093/oxfordhb/9780199739134.013.3

Beer, J. S., & Lombardo, M. V. (2009). Insight into emotion regulation from neuropsychology. In James J. Gross (Ed.), *Handbook of emotion regulation* (pp. 69–86). Guilford Press.

Berger, A. (2011). *Self-regulation: Brain, cognition and development*. American Psychological Association. https://doi.org/10.1037/12327-002

Bergeson, T. R., & Trehub, S. E. (2002). Absolute pitch and tempo in mothers' songs to infants. *Psychological Science, 13*(1), 72–75. https://doi.org/10.1111/1467-9280.00413

Bergman, K., Sarkar, P., Glover, V., & O'Connor, T. G. (2010). Maternal prenatal cortisol and infant cognitive development: Moderation by infant-mother attachment. *Biological Psychiatry, 67*(11), 1026–1032. https://doi.org/10.1016/j.biopsych.2010.01.002

Bezner Kerr, R., Dakishoni, L., Shumba, L., Msachi, R., & Chirwa, M. (2008). 'We grandmothers know plenty': Breastfeeding, complementary feeding and the multifaceted role of grandmothers in Malawi. *Social Science and Medicine, 66*(5), 1095–1105. https://doi.org/10.1016/j.socscimed.2007.11.019

Bieleninik, Ł., Ghetti, C., & Gold, C. (2016). Music therapy for preterm infants and their parents: A meta-analysis. *Pediatrics, 138*(3), e20160971. https://doi.org/10.1542/peds.2016-0971

Bieleninik, Ł., Konieczna-Nowak, L., Knapik-Szweda, S., & Kwaśniok, J. (2020). Evaluating feasibility of the LongSTEP (Longitudinal study of music therapy's effectiveness for premature infants and their caregivers) protocol with a Polish cohort. *Nordic Journal of Music Therapy, 29*(5), 437–459. https://doi.org/10.1080/08098131.2020.1781233

Bingley, K. (2011). Bambeh's Song: Music, women and health in a rural community in post-conflict Sierra Leone. *Music and Arts in Action, 3*(2), 59–78.

Blood, A. J., & Zatorre, R. J. (2001). Intensely pleasurable responses to music correlate with activity in brain regions implicated in reward and emotion. *Proceedings of the National Academy of Sciences of the United States of America, 98*(20), 11818–11823. https://doi.org/10.1073/pnas.191355898

Bohlman, P. V. (2002). *World music: A very short introduction*. Oxford University Press.

Braithwaite, E. C., Kundakovic, M., Ramchandani, P. G., Murphy, S. E., & Champagne, F. A. (2015). Maternal prenatal depressive symptoms predict infant NR3C1 1F and BDNF IV DNA methylation. *Epigenetics, 10*(5), 408–417. https://doi.org/10.1080/15592294.2015.1039221

Braungart-Rieker, J. M., Zentall, S., Lickenbrock, D. M., Ekas, N. V., Oshio, T., & Planalp, E. (2014). Attachment in the making: Mother and father sensitivity and infants' responses during the Still-Face Paradigm. *Journal of Experimental Child Psychology, 125*, 63–84. https://doi.org/10.1016/j.jecp.2014.02.007

Calkin, S. D., & Hill, A. (2007). Caregiver influences on biological and behavioral aspects of emotion regulation. In James J. Gross (Ed.), *Handbook of emotion regulation* (pp. 229–247). Guilford Press.

Cao, S., Sun, J., Wang, Y., Zhao, Y., Sheng, Y., & Xu, A. (2016). Music therapy improves pregnancy-induced hypertension treatment efficacy. *International Journal of Clinical and Experimental Medicine, 9*(5), 8833–8838. http://www.ijcem.com/files/ijcem0021741.pdf

Carral, V., Huotilainen, M., Ruusuvirta, T., Fellman, V., Näätänen, R., & Escera, C. (2005). A kind of auditory 'primitive intelligence' already present at birth. *European Journal of Neuroscience, 21*(11), 3201–3204. https://doi.org/10.1111/j.1460-9568.2005.04144.x

Carvajal, F., & Iglesias, J. (2006). Judgements of facial and vocal signs of emotion in infants with Down syndrome. *Developmental Psychobiology, 48*(8), 644–652. https://doi.org/10.1002/dev.20173

Cavaiuolo, C., Casani, A., Manso, D. G., & Orfeo, L. (2015). Effect of Mozart music on heel prick pain in preterm infants: A pilot randomized controlled trial. *Journal of Pediatric and Neonatal Individualized Medicine (JPNIM)*, 4(1), e040109. https://doi.org/10.7363/040109

Cevasco, A. M., & Grant, R. E. (2005). Effects of the pacifier activated lullaby on weight gain of premature infants. *Journal of Music Therapy*, 42(2), 123–139. https://doi.org/10.1093/jmt/42.2.123

Chang, H., Yu, C., Chen, S., & Chen, C. (2015). The effects of music listening on psychosocial stress and maternal–fetal attachment during pregnancy. *Complementary Therapies in Medicine*, 23(4), 509–515. https://doi.org/http://dx.doi.org/10.1016/j.ctim.2015.05.002

Chang, M.-Y., Chen, C.-H., & Huang, K.-F. (2008). Effects of music therapy on psychological health of women during pregnancy. *Journal of Clinical Nursing*, 17, 2580–2587. https://doi.org/10.1111/j.1365-2702.2007.02064.x

Chorna, O. D., Slaughter, J. C., Wang, L., Stark, A. R., & Maitre, N. L. (2014). A pacifier-activated music player with mother's voice improves oral feeding in preterm infants. *Pediatrics*, 133(3), 462–468. https://doi.org/10.1542/peds.2013-2547

Cicchetti, D., Ganiban, J., & Barnett, D. (1991). Contributions from the study of high-risk populations to understanding the development of emotion regulation. In J. Garber & K. A. Dodge (Eds.), *Cambridge studies in social and emotional development: The development of emotion regulation and dysregulation* (pp. 15–48). Cambridge University Press. https://doi.org/10.1017/CBO9780511663963.003

Cirelli, L. K., Einarson, K. M., & Trainor, L. J. (2014). Interpersonal synchrony increases prosocial behavior in infants. *Developmental Science*, 17(6), 1–9. https://doi.org/10.1111/desc.12193

Cirelli, L. K., & Trehub, S. E. (2018). Infants help singers of familiar songs. *Music & Science*, 1, 1–11. https://doi.org/10.1177/2059204318761622

Cirelli, L. K., Jurewicz, Z. B., & Trehub, S. E. (2019). Effects of maternal singing style on mother–infant arousal and behavior. *Journal of Cognitive Neuroscience*, 32(7), 1213–1220. https://doi.org/10.1162/jocn_a_01402

Cirelli, L. K., & Trehub, S. E. (2020). Familiar songs reduce infant distress. *Developmental Psychology*, 56(5), 861–868. https://doi.org/10.1037/dev0000917

Corbeil, M., Trehub, S. E., & Peretz, I. (2013). Speech vs. singing: Infants choose happier sounds. *Frontiers in Psychology*, 4, 372. https://doi.org/10.3389/fpsyg.2013.00372

Corbeil, M., Trehub, S. E., & Peretz, I. (2016). Singing delays the onset of infant distress. *Infancy*, 21(3), 373–391. https://doi.org/10.1111/infa.12114

Corrigall, K. A., & Trainor, L. J. (2014). Enculturation to musical pitch structure in young children: Evidence from behavioral and electrophysiological methods. *Developmental Science*, 17(1), 142–158. https://doi.org/10.1111/desc.12100

Costa-Giomi, E. (2014). Mode of presentation affects infants' preferential attention to singing and speech. *Music Perception*, 32(2), 160–169. https://doi.org/10.1525/mp.2014.32.2.160

Coyl, D. D., Roggman, L. A., & Newland, L. A. (2002). Stress, maternal depression, and negative mother-infant interactions in relation to infant attachment. *Infant Mental Health Journal*, 23(1–2), 145–163. https://doi.org/10.1002/imhj.10009

Cruz, M. D., Fernandes, A. M., & Oliveira, C. R. (2016). Epidemiology of painful procedures performed in neonates: A systematic review of observational studies. *European Journal of Pain*, 20(4), 489–498. https://doi.org/10.1002/ejp.757

de l'Etoile, S. K. (2006a). Infant behavioral responses to infant-directed singing and other maternal interactions. *Infant Behavior and Development*, 29(3), 456–470. https://doi.org/10.1016/j.infbeh.2006.03.002

de l'Etoile, S. K. (2006b). Infant-directed singing: A theory for clinical intervention. *Music Therapy Perspectives*, 24(1), 22–29. https://doi.org/10.1093/mtp/24.1.22

de l'Etoile, S. K. (2008). Teaching the youngest learners: Musical experiences for infants. *General Music Today, 22*(1), 35–37. https://doi.org/10.1177/1048371308323032

de l'Etoile, S. K. (2012). Responses to infant-directed singing in infants of mothers with depressive symptoms. *Arts in Psychotherapy, 39*(5), 353–366. https://doi.org/10.1016/j.aip.2012.05.003

de l'Etoile, S. K. (2015). Self-regulation and infant-directed singing in infants with Down syndrome. *Journal of Music Therapy, 52*(2), 195–220. https://doi.org/10.1093/jmt/thv003

de l'Etoile, S. K., & Leider, C. N. (2011). Acoustic parameters of infant-directed singing in mothers with depressive symptoms. *Infant Behavior and Development, 34*(2), 248–256. https://doi.org/10.1016/j.infbeh.2010.12.013

de l'Etoile, S. K., Behura, S., & Zopluoglu, C. (2017). Acoustic parameters of infant-directed singing in mothers of infants with Down syndrome. *Infant Behavior and Development, 49,* 151–160. https://doi.org/10.1016/j.infbeh.2017.09.001

de l'Etoile, S. K., Bennett, C., & Zopluoglu, C. (2020). Infant movement response to auditory rhythm. *Perceptual and Motor Skills, 127*(4), 651–670. https://doi.org/10.1177/0031512520922642

DeCasper, A. J., & Fifer, W. P. (1980). Of human bonding: Newborns prefer their mothers' voices. *Science, 208*(4448), 1174–1176. https://doi.org/10.1126/science.7375928

Donovan, W. L., Leavitt, L. A., & Walsh, R. O. (1998). Conflict and depression predict maternal sensitivity to infant cries. *Infant Behavior and Development, 21*(3), 505–517. https://doi.org/10.1016/S0163-6383(98)90023-6

Eckerdal, P., & Merker, B. (2009). 'Music' and the 'action song' in infant development: An interpretation. In C. Malloch & C. Trevarthen (Eds.), *Communicative musicality* (pp. 241–262). Oxford University Press.

Edwards, J. (2011). The use of music therapy to promote attachment between parents and infants. *Arts in Psychotherapy, 38*(3), 190–195. https://doi.org/10.1016/j.aip.2011.05.002

Ettenberger, M. (2017). Music therapy in the neonatal intensive care unit: Putting the families at the centre of care. *British Journal of Music Therapy, 31*(1), 12–17. https://doi.org/10.1177/1359457516685881

Fancourt, D., & Perkins, R. (2018). Effect of singing interventions on symptoms of postnatal depression: Three-arm randomised controlled trial. *British Journal of Psychiatry, 212,* 119–121. https://doi.org/10.1192/bjp.2017.29

Feldman, R. (2007). Parent-infant synchrony and the construction of shared timing: Physiological precursors, developmental outcomes, and risk conditions. *Journal of Child Psychology and Psychiatry, 48*(3–4), 329–354. https://doi.org/10.1111/j.1469-7610.2006.01701.x

Fifer, W., & Moon, C. (1994). The role of mother's voice in the organization of brain function in the newborn. *Acta Pædiatrica, 83*(s397), 86–93. https://doi.org/10.1111/j.1651-2227.1994.tb13270.x

Fisher, J., de Mello, M. C., Patel, V., Rahman, A., Tran, T., Holton, S., & Holmes, W. (2012). Prevalence and determinants of common perinatal mental disorders in women in low- and lower-middle-income countries: A systematic review. *Bulletin of the World Health Organization, 90,* 139–149. https://doi.org/10.2471/BLT.11.091850

Friedman, S. H., Kaplan, R. S., Rosenthal, M. B., & Console, P. (2010). Music therapy in perinatal psychiatry: Use of lullabies for pregnant and postpartum women with mental illness. *Music and Medicine, 2*(4), 219–225. https://doi.org/10.1177/1943862110379584

Gaden, T. S., Ghetti, C., Kvestad, I., & Gold, C. (2021). The LongSTEP approach: Theoretical framework and intervention protocol for using parent-driven infant-directed singing as resource-oriented music therapy. *Nordic Journal of Music Therapy,* 1–26. https://doi.org/10.1080/08098131.2021.1921014

Garunkstiene, R., Buinauskiene, J., Uloziene, I., & Markuniene, E. (2014). Controlled trial of live versus recorded lullabies in preterm infants. *Nordic Journal of Music Therapy*, *23*(1), 71–88. https://doi.org/10.1080/08098131.2013.809783

Ghazban, N. (2013). *Emotion regulation in infants using maternal singing and speech.* [Unpublished doctoral dissertation]. Ryerson University. https://rshare.library.ryerson.ca/

Ghetti, C. M., Bieleninik, Ł., Hysing, M., Kvestad, I., Assmus, J., Romeo, R., Ettenberger, M., Arnon, S., Vederhus, B. J., Gaden, T. S., & Gold, C. (2019). Longitudinal study of music therapy's effectiveness for premature infants and their caregivers (LongSTEP): Protocol for an international randomised trial. *BMJ Open*, *9*, e025062. https://doi.org/10.1136/bmjopen-2018-025062

Ghetti, C. M., Vederhus, B. J., Gaden, T. S., Brenner, A. K., Bieleninik, Ł., Kvestad, I., Assmus, J., & Gold, C. (2021). Longitudinal Study of music therapy's effectiveness for premature infants and their caregivers (LongSTEP): Feasibility study with a Norwegian cohort. *Journal of Music Therapy*, *58*(2), 201–240. https://doi.org/10.1093/jmt/thaa023

Glover, V. (2015). Prenatal stress and its effects on the fetus and the child: Possible underlying biological mechanisms. *Advances in Neurobiology*, *10*, 269–283. https://doi.org/10.1007/978-1-4939-1372-5_13

Glover, V, Bergman, K., Sarkar, P., & O'Connor, T. G. (2009). Association between maternal and amniotic fluid cortisol is moderated by maternal anxiety. *Psychoneuroendocrinology, 34*, 430–435. http://www.sciencedirect.com/science/article/pii/S0306453008002655

Glover, V., O'Connor, T. G., & O'Donnell, K. (2010). Prenatal stress and the programming of the HPA axis. *Neuroscience and Biobehavioral Reviews*, *35*(1)), 17–22. https://doi.org/10.1016/j.neubiorev.2009.11.008

Gooding, J. S., Cooper, L. G., Blaine, A. I., Franck, L. S., Howse, J. L., & Berns, S. D. (2011). Family support and family-centered care in the neonatal intensive care unit: Origins, advances, impact. *Seminars in Perinatology*, *35*(1), 20–28. https://doi.org/10.1053/j.semperi.2010.10.004

Gooding, L. F. (2010). Using music therapy protocols in the treatment of premature infants: An introduction to current practices. *Arts in Psychotherapy*, *37*(3), 211–214. https://doi.org/10.1016/j.aip.2010.04.003

Goodman, S. H., Radke-Yarrow, M., & Teti, D. (1993). Maternal depression as a context for child rearing. *Zero to Three*, *13*(5), 10–16.

Granier-Deferre, C., Bassereau, S., Ribeiro, A., Jacquet, A. Y., & DeCasper, A. J. (2011). A melodic contour repeatedly experienced by human near-term fetuses elicits a profound cardiac reaction one month after birth. *PLoS ONE*, *6*, e17304. https://doi.org/10.1371/journal.pone.0017304

Graven, S. N. (2000). Sound and the developing infant in the NICU: Conclusions and recommendations for care. *Journal of Perinatology*, *20*, s88–s93. https://doi.org/10.1038/sj.jp.7200444

Graven, S. N., & Browne, J. V. (2008). Auditory development in the fetus and infant. *Newborn and Infant Nursing Reviews*, *8*(4), 187–193. https://doi.org/10.1053/j.nainr.2008.10.010

Gross, J. J., & Thompson, R. A. (2007). Emotion regulation: Conceptual foundations. In J. J. Gross (Ed.), *Handbook of emotion regulation* (pp. 3–24). Guilford Press.

Gudmundsdottir, H., & Trehub, S. E. (2018). Adults recognize toddlers' song renditions. *Psychology of Music*, *46*(2), 281–291. https://doi.org/10.1177/0305735617711762

Háden, G. P., Honing, H., Török, M., & Winkler, I. (2015). Detecting the temporal structure of sound sequences in newborn infants. *International Journal of Psychophysiology*, *96*(1), 23–28. https://doi.org/10.1016/j.ijpsycho.2015.02.024

Hamm, E. L., Chorna, O. D., Flanery, A., & Maitre, N. L. (2017). A parent-infant music therapy intervention to improve neurodevelopment after neonatal intensive care. *Acta Pædiatrica*, *106*(10), 1703–1704. https://doi.org/10.1111/apa.13952

Hannon, E. E., & Trehub, S. E. (2005a). Metrical categories in infancy and adulthood. *Psychological Science, 16*(1), 48–55. https://doi.org/10.1111/j.0956-7976.2005.00779.x

Hannon, E. E., & Trehub, S. E. (2005b). Tuning in to musical rhythms: Infants learn more readily than adults. *Proceedings of the National Academy of Sciences, 102*(35), 12639–12643. https://doi.org/10.1073/pnas.0504254102

Haslbeck, F. B. (2012a). Music therapy for premature infants and their parents: An integrative review. *Nordic Journal of Music Therapy, 21*(3), 203–226. https://doi.org/10.1080/08098131.2011.648653

Haslbeck, F. B. (2012b). Research strategies to achieve a deeper understanding of active music therapy in neonatal care. *Music & Medicine, 4*(4), 205–214. https://doi.org/10.1177/1943862112458706

Heitmann, S., Faber, K., Kutz, P., Haus, R., & Roll, C. (2016). The effects of life music therapy on cerebral oxygenation and on vital signs in preterm infants. *European Journal of Pediatrics, 175*(11), 1707. https://doi.org/10.1007/s00431-016-2785-8

Hepper, P. G. (1991). An examination of fetal learning before and after birth. *The Irish Journal of Psychology, 12*(2), 95–107. https://doi.org/10.1080/03033910.1991.10557830

Hepper, P. G., Scott, D., & Shahidullah, S. (1993). Newborn and fetal response to maternal voice. *Journal of Reproductive and Infant Psychology, 11*(3), 147–153. https://doi.org/10.1080/02646839308403210

Hepper, P. G., & Shahidullah, B. S. (1994). The development of fetal hearing. *Fetal and Maternal Medicine Review, 6*(3), 167–179. https://doi.org/10.1017/S0965539500001108

Hugh, S. C., Wolter, N. E., Propst, E. J., Gordon, K. A., Cushing, S. L., & Papsin, B. C. (2014). Infant sleep machines and hazardous sound pressure levels. *Pediatrics, 133*(4), 677–681. https://doi.org/10.1542/peds.2013-3617

Hunziker, U. A., & Barr, R. G. (1986). Increased carrying reduces infant crying: A randomized controlled trial. *Pediatrics, 77*(5), 641–648. https://www.researchgate.net/publication/19643720

Ilari, B., Moura, A., & Bourscheidt, L. (2011). Between interactions and commodities: Musical parenting of infants and toddlers in Brazil. *Music Education Research, 13*(1), 51–67. https://doi.org/10.1080/14613808.2011.553277

Jahn, M., Müller-Mazzotta, J., & Arabin, B. (2016). Music devices for the fetus? An evaluation of pregnancy music belts. *Journal of Perinatal Medicine, 44*(6), 637–643. https://doi.org/10.1515/jpm-2015-0074

Jernigan, T. L., Bellugi, U., Sowell, E., Doherty, S., & Hesselink, J. R. (1993). Cerebral morphologic distinctions between Williams and Down syndromes. *Archives of Neurology, 50*(2), 186–191. https://doi.org/10.1001/archneur.1993.00540020062019

Kafali, H., Derbent, A., Keskin, E., Simavli, S., & Gozdemir, E. (2011). Effect of maternal anxiety and music on fetal movements and fetal heart rate patterns. *The Journal of Maternal-Fetal and Neonatal Medicine, 24*(3), 461–464. https://doi.org/10.3109/14767058.2010.501122

Keith, D. R., Russell, K., & Weaver, B. S. (2009). The effects of music listening on incosolable crying in premature infants. *Journal of Music Therapy, 46*(3), 191–203. https://doi.org/10.1093/jmt/46.3.191

Kogan, M. D., Kotelchuck, M., Alexander, G. R., & Johnson, W. E. (1994). Racial disparities in reported prenatal care advice from health care providers. *American Journal of Public Health, 84*(1), 82–88. https://doi.org/10.2105/AJPH.84.1.82

Lassi, Z., & Bhutta, Z. (2015). Community-based intervention packages for reducing maternal and neonatal morbidity and mortality and improving neonatal outcomes. *Cochrane Database of Systematic Reviews, 3.* https://doi.org/10.1002/14651858.CD007754.pub3

Lecanuet, J.-P. (1996). Prenatal auditory experience. In I. Deliège & J. A. Sloboda (Eds.), *Musical beginnings: Origins and development of musical competence* (pp. 45–66). Oxford University Press. https://doi.org/10.1093/acprof

Leerkes, E. M., Nayena Blankson, A., & O'Brien, M. (2009). Differential effects of maternal sensitivity to infant distress and nondistress on social-emotional functionin. *Child Development, 80*(3), 762–775. https://doi.org/10.1111/j.1467-8624.2009.01296.x

LeVine, R. A. (1988). Human parental care: Universal goals, cultural strategies, individual behavior. *New Directions for Child and Adolescent Development, 1988*(40), 3–12. https://doi.org/10.1002/cd.23219884003

Lillas, C., & Turnbull, J. (2009). *Infant/child mental health, early intervention, and relationship-based therapies: A neurorelational framework for interdisciplinary practice.* W. W. Norton. https://books.google.com/books?hl=en&lr=&id=Y2qaKXZu6EsC&oi=fnd&pg=PR25&dq=interdisciplinary+challenges+infant+music+therapy&ots=9cwXjjM-AM&sig=0MNh18KDXv4qOxD5nb3hWxm6mBg

Loewy, J. (2015). NICU music therapy: Song of kin as critical lullaby in research and practice. *Annals of the New York Academy of Sciences, 1337*(1), 178–185. https://doi.org/10.1111/nyas.12648

Loewy, J., Stewart, K., Dassler, A.-M., Telsey, A., & Homel, P. (2013). The effects of music therapy on vital signs, feeding, and sleep in premature infants. *Pediatrics, 131*(5), 902–918. https://doi.org/10.1542/peds.2012-1367

Lu, M. C., & Halfon, N. (2003). Racial and ethnic disparities in birth outcomes: A life-course perspective. *Maternal and Child Health Journal, 7*(1), 13–30. https://doi.org/10.1023/A:1022537516969

Malloch, S. N. (1999). Mothers and infants and communicative musicality. *Musicae Scientiae, 3*(1 suppl.), 29–57. https://doi.org/10.1177/10298649000030S104

Malloch, S. N., & Trevarthen, C. (2009). Musicality: Communicating the vitality and interests of life. In S. Malloch & C. Trevarthen (Eds.), *Communicative musicality: Exploring the basis of human companionship* (pp. 1–11). Oxford University Press.

Malloch, S. N., Shoemark, H., Črnčec, R., Newnham, C., Paul, C., Prior, M., Coward, S., & Burnham, D. (2012). Music therapy with hospitalized infants—The art and science of communicative musicality. *Infant Mental Health Journal, 33*(4), 386–399. https://doi.org/10.1002/imhj.21346

Margulis, E. H. (2014). *On repeat: How music plays the mind.* Oxford University Press.

Marwick, H., & Murray, L. (2009). The effects of maternal depression on the 'musicality' of infant-directed speech and conversational engagement. In S. Malloch & C. Trevarthen (Eds.), *Communicative musicality: Exploring the basis of human companionship.* (pp. 281–300). Oxford University Press. https://strathprints.strath.ac.uk/id/eprint/26400

Masataka, N. (1999). Preference for infant-directed singing in 2-day-old hearing infants of deaf parents. *Developmental Psychology, 35*(4), 1001–1005. https://doi.org/10.1037/0012-1649.35.4.1001

McConnell, B. B. (2015). *Singing the unsayable: Female performers and global health in The Gambia.* [Unpublished doctoral dissertation] University of Washington. https://digital.lib.washington.edu/researchworks/handle/1773/34084

McConnell, B. B. (2016). Music and health communication in The Gambia: A social capital approach. *Social Science and Medicine, 169*, 132–140. https://doi.org/10.1016/j.socscimed.2016.09.028

McConnell, B. B. (2017). Performing 'participation': Kanyeleng musicians and global health in The Gambia. *Ethnomusicology, 61*(2), 312–332.

McConnell, B. B. (2020). *Music, health, and power: Singing the unsayable in The Gambia.* Routledge. https://doi.org/10.4324/9780367312732

McLean, E., McFerran, K. S., & Thompson, G. A. (2019). Parents' musical engagement with their baby in the neonatal unit to support emerging parental identity: A grounded theory study. *Journal of Neonatal Nursing, 25*(2), 78–85. https://doi.org/10.1016/j.jnn.2018.09.005

Meenakshi, S. (2016). A quasi experimental study to assess the effectiveness of music therapy on stress and blood pressure among antenatal mothers with Pregnancy Induced Hypertension at selected hospitals of Punjab. *International Journal of Advances in Nursing Management*, *4*(4), 355–360. https://doi.org/10.5958/2454-2652.2016.00079.2

Mehr, S. A., Song, L. A., & Spelke, E. S. (2016). For 5-month-old infants, melodies are social. *Psychological Science*, *27*(4), 486–501. https://doi.org/10.1177/0956797615626691

Mehr, S. A., Singh, M., York, H., Glowacki, L., & Krasnow, M. M. (2018). Form and function in human song. *Current Biology*, *28*(3), 356–368. https://doi.org/10.1016/j.cub.2017.12.042

Mehr, S. A., Singh, M., Knox, D., Ketter, D. M., Pickens-Jones, D., Atwood, S., Lucas, C., Jacoby, N., Egner, A. A., Hopkins, E. J., Howard, R. M., Hartshorne, J. K., Jennings, M. V., Simson, J., Bainbridge, C. M., Pinker, S., O'Donnell, T. J., Krasnow, M. M., & Glowacki, L. (2019). Universality and diversity in human song. *Science*, *366*(6468), eaax0868. https://doi.org/10.1126/science.aax0868

Menon, V., & Levitin, D. J. (2005). The rewards of music listening: Response and physiological connectivity of the mesolimbic system. *NeuroImage*, *28*(1), 175–184. https://doi.org/10.1016/j.neuroimage.2005.05.053

Milgrom, J., Gemmill, A. W., Bilszta, J. L., Hayes, B., Barnett, B., Brooks, J., Ericksen, J., Ellwood, D., & Buist, A. (2008). Antenatal risk factors for postnatal depression: A large prospective study. *Journal of Affective Disorders*, *108*(1–2), 147–157. https://doi.org/10.1016/j.jad.2007.10.014

Milligan, K., Atkinson, L., Trehub, S. E., Benoit, D., & Poulton, L. (2003). Maternal attachment and the communication of emotion through song. *Infant Behavior and Development*, *26*(1), 1–13. https://doi.org/10.1016/S0163-6383(02)00165-0

Moon, C. (2017). Prenatal experience with the maternal voice. In M. Filippa, P. Kuhn, & B. Westrup (Eds.), *Early vocal contact and preterm infant brain development* (pp. 25–37). Springer; Cham. https://doi.org/10.1007/978-3-319-65077-7_2

Moore, D., Oates, J., Goodwin, J., & Hobson, R. P. (2008). Behavior of mothers and infants with and without Down syndrome during the still-face procedure. *Infancy*, *13*(1), 75–89. https://doi.org/10.1080/15250000701779394

Morelli, G. A., Rogoff, B., Oppenheim, D., & Goldsmith, D. (1992). Cultural variation in infants' sleeping arrangements: Questions of independence. *Developmental Psychology*, *28*(4), 604–613. https://doi.org/10.1037/0012-1649.28.4.604

Murray, L., Fiori-Cowley, A., Hooper, R., & Cooper, P. (1996). The impact of postnatal depression and associated adversity on early mother-infant interactions and later infant outcome. *Child Development*, *67*(5), 2512–2526. https://doi.org/10.2307/1131637

Nakata, T., & Trehub, S. E. (2004). Infants' responsiveness to maternal speech and singing. *Infant Behavior and Development*, *27*(4), 455–464. https://doi.org/10.1016/j.infbeh.2004.03.002

Nakata, T., & Trehub, S. E. (2011). Expressive timing and dynamics in infant-directed and non-infant-directed singing. *Psychomusicology: Music, Mind and Brain*, *21*(1–2), 130–138. https://doi.org/10.1037/h0094003

Nicholson, J. M., Berthelsen, D., Abad, V., Williams, K., & Bradley, J. (2008). Impact of music therapy to promote positive parenting and child development. *Journal of Health Psychology*, *13*(2), 226–238. https://doi.org/10.1177/1359105307086705

Nwebube, C., Glover, V., & Stewart, L. (2017). Prenatal listening to songs composed for pregnancy and symptoms of anxiety and depression: A pilot study. *BMC Complementary and Alternative Medicine*, *17*, 256. https://doi.org/10.1186/s12906-017-1759-3

O'Gorman, S. (2007). Infant-directed singing in neonatal and paediatric intensive care. *Australian and New Zealand Journal of Family Therapy*, *28*(2), 100–108. https://doi.org/10.1375/anft.28.2.100

O'Toole, A., Francis, K., & Pugsley, L. (2017). Does music positively impact preterm infant outcomes? *Advances in Neonatal Care*, *17*(3), 192–202. https://doi.org/10.1097/ANC.0000000000000394

Oh, M. O., Kim, Y. J., Baek, C. H., Kim, J. H., Park, N. M., Yu, M. J., & Song, H. S. (2016). Effect of music intervention on maternal anxiety and fetal heart rate pattern during non-stress test. *Journal of Korean Academy of Nursing, 46*(3), 315–326. https://doi.org/10.4040/jkan.2016.46.3.315

Olischar, M., Shoemark, H., Holton, T., Weninger, M., & Hunt, R. W. (2011). The influence of music on aEEG-activity in neurologically healthy newborns > 32 weeks' gestational age. *Acta Pædiatrica, 100*(5), 670–675. https://doi.org/10.1111/j.1651-2227.2011.02171.x

Owens, J. A. (2004). Sleep in children: Cross-cultural perspectives. *Sleep and Biological Rhythms, 2*(3), 165–173. https://doi.org/10.1111/j.1479-8425.2004.00147.x

Palazzi, A., Nunes, C. C., & Piccinini, C. A. (2018). Music therapy and musical stimulation in the context of prematurity: A narrative literature review from 2010–2015. *Journal of Clinical Nursing, 27*(1–2), e1–e20. https://doi.org/10.1111/jocn.13893

Pantaleoni, H. (1985). *On the nature of music.* Welkin.

Parncutt, R. (2016). Prenatal development. In G. E. McPherson (Ed.), *The child as musician: A handbook of musical development* (2nd ed., pp. 3–31). Oxford University Press.

Payne, C., & Bachevalier, J. (2009). Neuroanatomy of the developing social brain. In M. De Haan, & M. R. Gunnar (Eds.), *Handbook of developmental social neuroscience* (pp. 38–59). Guilford Press.

Perkins, R., Yorke, S., & Fancourt, D. (2018). How group singing facilitates recovery from the symptoms of postnatal depression: A comparative qualitative study. *BMC Psychology, 6*, 41. https://doi.org/10.1186/s40359-018-0253-0

Persico, G., Antolini, L., Vergani, P., Costantini, W., Nardi, M. T., & Bellotti, L. (2017). Maternal singing of lullabies during pregnancy and after birth: Effects on mother–infant bonding and on newborns' behaviour. Concurrent Cohort Study. *Women and Birth.* https://doi.org/10.1016/j.wombi.2017.01.007

Phillips-Silver, J., & Trainor, L. J. (2005). Feeling the beat: Movement influences infant rhythm perception. *Science, 308*(5727), 1430. https://doi.org/10.1126/science.1110922

Pickett, K. E., Shaw, R. J., Atkin, K., Kiernan, K. E., & Wilkinson, R. G. (2009). Ethnic density effects on maternal and infant health in the Millennium Cohort Study. *Social Science and Medicine, 69*(10), 1476–1483. https://doi.org/10.1016/j.socscimed.2009.08.031

Pineda, R., Guth, R., Herring, A., Reynolds, L., Oberle, S., & Smith, J. (2017). Enhancing sensory experiences for very preterm infants in the NICU: An integrative review. *Journal of Perinatology, 37*(4), 323–332). https://doi.org/10.1038/jp.2016.179

Pinter, J. D., Brown, W. E., Eliez, S., Schmitt, J. E., Capone, G. T., & Reiss, A. L. (2001). Amygdala and hippocampal volumes in children with Down syndrome: A high- resolution MRI study. *Neurology, 56*(7), 972–974. https://doi.org/10.1212/WNL.56.7.972

Plantinga, J., & Trainor, L. J. (2005). Memory for melody: Infants use a relative pitch code. *Cognition, 98*(1), 1–11. https://doi.org/10.1016/j.cognition.2004.09.008

Pound, G. A. (2005). *The relationship between postpartum depression and infant development* [Unpublished doctoral dissertation]. California School of Professional Psychology. https://www.proquest.com/dissertations-theses/relationship-between-postpartum-depression-in-fant/docview/304909888/se-2?accountid=14511

Prost, A., Colbourn, T., Seward, N., Azad, K., Coomarasamy, A., Copas, A., Houweling, T. A. J., Fottrell, E., Kuddus, A., Lewycka, S., MacArthur, C., Manandhar, D., Morrison, J., Mwansambo, C., Nair, N., Nambiar, B., Osrin, D., Pagel, C., Phiri, T., . . . Costello, A. (2013). Women's groups practising participatory learning and action to improve maternal and new-born health in low-resource settings: A systematic review and meta-analysis. *Lancet, 381*, 1736–1746. https://doi.org/10.1016/S0140-6736(13)60685-6

Quadros, A. de, & Dorstewitz, P. (2011). Community, communication, social change: Music in dispossessed Indian communities. *International Journal of Community Music, 4*(1), 59–70. https://doi.org/10.1386/ijcm.4.1.59_1

Querleu, D., Lefebvre, C., Titran, M., Renard, X., Morillion, M., & Crepin, G. (1984). Reaction of the newborn infant less than 2 hours after birth to the maternal voice. *Journal de Gynécologie Obstetrique et Biologie de la Réproduction*, *13*(2), 125–134. http://europepmc.org/abstract/med/6736589

Querleu, D., Renard, X., Versyp, F., Paris-Delrue, L., & Crèpin, G. (1988). Fetal hearing. *European Journal of Obstetrics and Gynecology and Reproductive Biology*, *28*(3), 191–212. https://doi.org/10.1016/0028-2243(88)90030-5

Rahman, A., Surkan, P. J., Cayetano, C. E., Rwagatare, P., & Dickson, K. E. (2013). Grand mhallenges: Integrating maternal mental health into maternal and child health programmes. *PLOS Medicine*, *10*(5). https://doi.org/10.1371/journal.pmed.1001442:

Robertson, E., Grace, S., Wallington, T., & Stewart, D. E. (2004). Antenatal risk factors for postpartum depression: A synthesis of recent literature. *General Hospital Psychiatry*, *26*, 289–295. https://doi.org/10.1016/j.genhosppsych.2004.02.006

Rothbaum, F., Pott, M., Azuma, H., Miyake, K., & Weisz, J. (2000). The development of close relationships in Japan and the United States: Paths of symbiotic harmony and generative tension. *Child Development*, *71*(5), 1121–1142. https://doi.org/10.1111/1467-8624.00214

Sanfilippo, K. R. M. (2020). *Developing a community-led music intervention to support antenatal mental health in The Gambia*. [Unpublished doctoral dissertation].Goldsmiths, University of London. https://research.gold.ac.uk/id/eprint/30166/

Sanfilippo, K. R. M., McConnell, B., Cornelius, V., Darboe, B., Huma, H. B., Gaye, M., Ceesay, H., Ramchandani, P., Cross, I., Glover, V., & Stewart, L. (2020). Community psychosocial music intervention (CHIME) to reduce antenatal common mental disorder symptoms in The Gambia: a feasibility trial. *BMJ Open*, *10*(11), e040287. https://doi.org/10.1136/bmjopen-2020-040287

Savage, P. E., Brown, S., Sakai, E., & Currie, T. E. (2015). Statistical universals reveal the structures and functions of human music. *Proceedings of the National Academy of Sciences of the United States*, *112*(29), 8987–8992. https://doi.org/10.1073/pnas.1414495112

Schäfer, K., Saarikallio, S., & Eerola, T. (2020). Music may reduce loneliness and act as social surrogate for a friend: Evidence from an experimental listening study. *Music & Science*, *3*, 1–16. https://doi.org/10.1177/2059204320935709

Schetter, C. D., & Glynn, L. M. (2010). Stress in pregnancy: Empirical evidence and theoretical issues to guild interdisciplinary research. In R. J. Contrada & A. Baum (Eds.), *The handbook of stress science: Biology, psychology, and health* (pp. 321–347). Springer Publishing.

Schlez, A., Litmanovitz, I., Bauer, S., Dolfin, T., Regev, R., & Arnon, S. (2011). Combining kangaroo care and live harp music therapy in the neonatal intensive care unit setting. *Israel Medical Association Journal*, *13*(6), 354–358. https://www.ima.org.il/imaj/viewarticle.aspx-?year=2011&month=06&page=354

Schore, A. N. (2000). Attachment and the regulation of the right brain. *Attachment and Human Development*, *2*(1), 23–47. https://doi.org/10.1080/146167300361309

Shenfield, T., Trehub, S. E., & Nakata, T. (2003). Maternal singing modulates infant arousal. *Psychology of Music*, *31*(4), 365–375. https://doi.org/10.1177/03057356030314002

Shin, H. S., & Kim, J. H. (2011). Music therapy on anxiety, stress and maternal-fetal attachment in pregnant women during transvaginal ultrasound. *Asian Nursing Research*, *5*(1), 19–27. https://doi.org/10.1016/S1976-1317(11)60010-8

Shoemark, H., & Dearn, T. (2008). Keeping parents at the centre of family centred music therapy with hospitalised infants. *The Australian Journal of Music Therapy*, *19*, 3–26. http://search.proquest.com/openview/c909d1dd4143cb14/1.pdf?pq-origsite=gscholar&cbl=13373

Shoemark, H., & Grocke, D. (2010). The markers of interplay between the music therapist and the high risk full term infant. *Journal of Music Therapy*, *47*(4), 306–334. https://doi.org/10.1093/jmt/47.4.306

Shoemark, H., & Ettenberger, M. (Eds.). (2020). *Music therapy in neonatal intensive care: Influences of culture*. Barcelona Publishers.

Shoemark, H., Hanson-Abromeit, D., & Stewart, L. (2015). Constructing optimal experience for the hospitalized newborn through neuro-based music therapy. *Frontiers in Human Neuroscience, 9*, 487. https://doi.org/10.3389/fnhum.2015.00487

Silver, D. (2001). Songs and storytelling: Bringing health messages to life in Uganda. *Education for Health, 14*(1), 51–60. https://doi.org/10.1080/13576280010015362

Skramstad, H. (2008). *Making and managing femaleness, fertility and motherhood within an urban Gambian area.* [Unpublished doctoral dissertation].University of Bergen. https://bora.uib.no/bora-xmlui/handle/1956/2737

Slonims, V., & McConachie, H. (2006). Analysis of mother–infant interaction in infants with Down syndrome and typically developing infants. *American Journal of Mental Retardation, 111*(4), 273–289. https://doi.org/10.1352/0895-8017(2006)111[273:AOMIII]2.0.CO;2

Sole, M. (2017). Crib song: Insights into functions of toddlers' private spontaneous singing. *Psychology of Music, 45*(2), 172–192. https://doi.org/10.1177/0305735616650746

Speranza, A. M., Ammaniti, M., & Trentini, C. (2006). An overview of maternal depression, infant reactions and intervention programmes. *Clinical Neurophysiology, 3*(1), 57–68. https://www.researchgate.net/profile/Cristina_Trentini/publication/257937624_An_overview_of_maternal_depression_Infant_reactions_and_intervention_programmes/links/0c96052658a5426f1c000000.pdf

Spiker, D. (2006). Off to a good start: Early intervention for infants and young children with Down syndrome and their families. In J. A. Rondal & J. Perera (Eds.), *Down syndrome: Neurobehavioral specificity* (pp. 175–190). John Wiley & Sons.

Sroufe, L. A. (2000). Early relationships and the development of children. *Infant Mental Health Journal, 21*(1–2), 67–74. https://doi.org/10.1002/(SICI)1097-0355(200001/04)21:1/2<67::AID-IMHJ8>3.0.CO;2-2

Standley, J. M. (1991). The role of music in pacification/stimulation of premature infants with low birthweights. *Music Therapy Perspectives, 9*(1), 19–25. https://doi.org/10.1093/mtp/9.1.19

Standley, J. M. (1998). The effect of music and multimodal stimulation on responses of premature infants in neonatal intensive care. *Pediatric Nursing, 24*(6), 532–538. http://search.proquest.com/openview/16b96431ffbe800457f284a34ffa20a3/1?pq-origsite=gscholar&cbl=47659

Standley, J. M., & Whipple, J. (2003). Music therapy for premature infants in the neonatal intensive care unit: Health and developmental benefits. In S. L. Robb (Ed.), *Music therapy in pediatric healthcare: Research and evidence-based practice* (pp. 19–30). American Music Therapy Association.

Terry, M. M., & Terry, D. R. (2012). Singing the blues: A literature review of the effects of music on postnatal depression. *International Journal of Innovative Interdisciplinary, 1*(3), 55–67.

Thompson, R. A. (1994). Emotion regulation: A theme in search of definition. *Monographs of the Society for Research in Child Developmen, 59*(2–3), 25–52. http://onlinelibrary.wiley.com/doi/10.1111/j.1540-5834.1994.tb01276.x/full

Trainor, L. J. (1996). Infant preferences for infant-directed versus noninfant-directed playsongs and lullabies. *Infant Behavior and Development, 19*(1), 83–92. https://doi.org/10.1016/S0163-6383(96)90046-6

Trehub, S. E. (2016). Infant musicality. In S. Hallam, I. Cross, & M. Thaut (Eds.), *The Oxford handbook of music psychology* (2nd ed., pp. 387–398). Oxford University Press. https://doi.org/10.1093/oxfordhb/9780198722946.013.26

Trehub, S. E., Unyk, A. M., & Trainor, L. J. (1993). Maternal singing in cross-cultural perspective. *Journal of Infant Behavior & Development, 16*(3), 285–295. https://www.sciencedirect.com/science/article/pii/0163638393800368

Trehub, S. E., Unyk, A. M., Kamenetsky, S. B., Hill, D. S., Trainor, L. J., Henderson, J. L., & Saraza, M. (1997). Mothers' and fathers' singing to infants. *Developmental Psychology, 33*(3), 500–507. https://doi.org/http://dx.doi.org/10.1037/0012-1649.33.3.500

Trehub, S. E., & Trainor, L. (1998). Singing to infants: Lullabies and play songs. *Advances in Infancy Research, 12*, 43–77.

Trehub, S. E., & Prince, R. (2010). Lullabies and other women's songs in the Turkish village of Akçaeniş. *UNESCO Observatory E-Journal, 2*(2), 1–19.

Trehub, S. E., Ghazban, N., & Corbeil, M. (2015). Musical affect regulation in infancy. *Annals of the New York Academy of Sciences, 1337*, 186–192. https://doi.org/10.1111/nyas.12622

Trehub, S. E., & Gudmundsdottir, H. R. (2019). Mothers as singing mentors for infants. In G. F. Welch, J. Nix, & D. Howard (Eds.), *The Oxford handbook of singing* (pp. 455–469). Oxford University Press. https://doi.org/10.1093/oxfordhb/9780199660773.013.25

Trehub, S. E., Plantinga, J., & Russo, F. A. (2016). Maternal vocal interactions with infants: Reciprocal visual influences. *Social Development, 25*(3), 665–683. https://doi.org/10.1111/sode.12164

Trehub, S. E., & Russo, F. A. (2020). Infant-directed singing from a dynamic multimodal perspective: Evolutionary origins, cross-cultural variation, and relation to infant-directed speech. In F. A. Russo, B. Ilari, & A. J. Cohen (Eds.), *The Routledge companion to interdisciplinary studies in singing. Vol. I. Development* (pp. 249–261). Routledge.

Ullsten, A., Eriksson, M., Klässbo, M., & Volgsten, U. (2016). Live music therapy with lullaby singing during painful procedures in neonatal care. *Nordic Journal of Music Therapy, 25*(sup1), 79. http://www.diva-portal.org/smash/record.jsf?pid=diva2:951202

van der Heijden, M. J. E., Oliai Araghi, S., Jeekel, J., Reiss, I. K. M., Hunink, M. G. M., & van Dijk, M. (2016). Do hospitalized premature infants benefit from music interventions? A systematic review of randomized controlled trials. *PLOS ONE, 11*(9), e0161848. https://doi.org/10.1371/journal.pone.0161848

van Puyvelde, M., Loots, G., Vinck, B., De Coster, L., Matthijs, L., Mouvet, K., & Pattyn, N. (2013). The interplay between tonal synchrony and social engagement in mother-infant interaction. *Infancy, 18*(5), 849–872. https://doi.org/10.1111/infa.12007

van Puyvelde, M., Rodrigues, H., Loots, G., De Coster, L., Du Ville, K., Matthijs, L., Simcock, D., & Pattyn, N. (2014). Shall we dance? Music as a port of entrance to maternal-infant intersubjectivity in a context of postnatal depression. *Infant Mental Health Journal, 35*(3), 220–232. https://doi.org/10.1002/imhj.21431

Vohs, K. D., & Baumeister, R. F. (2004). Understanding self-regulation: An introduction. In R. F. Baumeister & K. D. Vohs (Eds.), *Handbook of self-regulation: Research, theory, and applications* (pp. 1–9). Guilford Press.

Volkova, A., Trehub, S. E., & Glenn Schellenberg, E. (2006). Infants' memory for musical performances. *Developmental Science, 9*(6), 583–589. https://doi.org/10.1111/j.1467-7687.2006.00536.x

Walworth, D. D. (2009). Effects of developmental music groups for parents and premature or typical infants under two years on parental responsiveness and infant social development. *Journal of Music Therapy, 46*(1), 32–52. https://doi.org/10.1093/jmt/46.1.32

Wheeler, B. L., & Stultz, S. (2008). Using typical infant development to inform music therapy with children with disabilities. *Early Childhood Education Journal, 35*(6), 585–591. https://doi.org/10.1007/s10643-007-0224-1

Whipple, J. (2000). The effect of parent training in music and multimodal stimulation on parent-neonate interactions in the neonatal intensive care unit. *Journal of Music Therapy, 37*(4), 250–268. https://doi.org/10.1093/jmt/37.4.250

Williams, K. E., Berthelsen, D., Nicholson, J. M., Walker, S., & Abad, V. (2012). The effectiveness of a short-term group music therapy intervention for parents who have a child with a disability. *Journal of Music Therapy, 49*(1), 23–44. https://doi.org/10.1093/jmt/49.1.23

Winkler, I., Haden, G. P., Ladinig, O., Sziller, I., & Honing, H. (2009). Newborn infants detect the beat in music. *Proceedings of the National Academy of Sciences of the United States*, *106*(7), 2468–2471. https://doi.org/10.1073/pnas.0809035106

World Health Organization. (2015). Health in 2015: From MDGs, millennium development goals to SDGs, sustainable development goals. In *World Health Organisation*. https://doi. org/978 92 4 156511 0

Wulff, V., Hepp, P., Fehm, T., & Schaal, N. (2017). Music in obstetrics: An intervention option to reduce tension, pain and stress. *Geburtshilfe und Frauenheilkunde*, *77*, 967–975. https:// doi.org/10.1055/s-0043-118414

Wulff, V., Hepp, P., Wolf, O. T., Balan, P., Hagenbeck, C., Fehm, T., & Schaal, N. K. (2021). The effects of a music and singing intervention during pregnancy on maternal well-being and mother–infant bonding: A randomised, controlled study. *Archives of Gynecology and Obstetrics*, *303*(1), 69–83. https://doi.org/10.1007/s00404-020-05727-8

Zentner, M., & Eerola, T. (2010). Rhythmic engagement with music in infancy. *Proceedings of the National Academy of Sciences of the United States*, *107*(13), 5768–5773. https://doi.org/ 10.1073/pnas.1000121107

Zimmer, E. Z., Divon, M. Y., Vilensky, A., Sarna, Z., Peretz, B. A., & Paldi, E. (1982). Maternal exposure to music and fetal activity. *European Journal of Obstetrics and Gynecology and Reproductive Biology*, *13*(4), 209–213. https://doi.org/10.1016/0028-2243(82)90101-0

2

Musical care in childhood

How music nurtures the developing child

Camilla Farrant, Tal-Chen Rabinowitch, and Nicola Dunbar

Introduction

Music has multiple roles in the nurturing of a child. From the individual to the social to the community, music can have a powerful impact, influencing children's emotions, behaviour, and cognition through a variety of music activities. This chapter touches upon the potential that music has to simultaneously nurture children intellectually, physically, socially, and emotionally.

Music is a lively, dynamic, and engaging art form, an expressive tool for human communication and an instrument for caregiving. As discussed in the Musical care in infancy chapter, music is inherent in the exaggerated rhythmicity and prosody of infant-directed speech (Bergeson & Trehub, 2007; Fernald et al., 1989), and in the melodic contours of their vocalizations (Papoušek, 1996; Papoušek & Papoušek, 1981). Moreover, as children get older, their capacity for musicality, musical engagement, and musical skill develops (Lamont, 2009). From listening to music on the radio and singing and dancing in the playground, to some children even learning how to play an instrument, music plays an intrinsic part in the all-round care of a child as they experience the world around them. Musical care, in this chapter, refers to the ability music has to nurture a child's development in a multitude of areas.

We focus on the ages 5 to 12 years; a period of middle childhood that typically encompasses rapid developmental change (Piaget & Inhelder, 2008; Shaffer, 2013). Many studies we reference also discuss children just outside this age bracket, yet we try to focus on the range of developmental characteristics typically associated with this stage of childhood; namely, rapid intellectual, physical, social, and emotional growth (Papalia et al., 2007). We use the term 'nurture' to evoke the idea that music can be used as an action with consequences—an act of caregiving that influences the quality of a child's development.

Mirroring the vast range of ways in which music nurtures childhood, this chapter provides an interdisciplinary overview of musical care in childhood through drawing together the authors' research and clinical knowledge. As practitioners and researchers, we each represent and bridge the worlds of music therapy, music education, and music psychology. Camilla Farrant is a music therapy practitioner-researcher,

Camilla Farrant, Tal-Chen Rabinowitch, and Nicola Dunbar, *Musical care in childhood* In: *Collaborative Insights.*
Edited by: Neta Spiro and Katie Rose M. Sanfilippo, Oxford University Press. © Oxford University Press 2022.
DOI: 10.1093/oso/9780197535011.003.0003

Tal-Chen Rabinowitch is a researcher in music education and music psychology with experience in teaching and music interventions, and Nicola Dunbar is a music therapist and child and family psychotherapist. To complement the cross-disciplinary research studies explored in this chapter, each section ends with a vignette from music therapy practice to bring to life how music can directly nurture or influence a child's development.

Much engagement in music—such as listening to music through headphones or attending a concert—can be seen as a *passive* mode of entertainment. However, this notion of passivity can be misleading even when it comes to music listening. Previous studies have shown that listening to music evokes strong emotional reactions (Juslin & Sloboda, 2001) and engages motor cortical areas (Zatorre et al., 2007) involved in supporting voluntary movements. When we are listening to music it is hard to resist the urge to respond through movement and most of us can testify to feeling emotionally moved when hearing a particular piece or song (Juslin & Sloboda, 2001). Findings from neuroscience have suggested that when we are observing someone else perform an action, areas of the brain involved in performing that action are activated even though we are not physically performing that action ourselves (Iacoboni et al., 1999)—this 'mirroring' process activates the mirror neuron system. The mirror neuron system has been suggested as a mechanism that may explain why we feel compelled to move or emotionally respond when we listen to some music (Koelsch et al., 2006; Molnar-Szakacs & Overy, 2006). For instance, when we watch or simply hear someone play an instrument, the neurons in the brain that are associated with the muscles required to perform that action are active, just as if we were performing ourselves, not merely listening (Keysers et al., 2003; Kohler et al., 2002; Rizzolatti & Craighero, 2004; Watkins et al., 2003). Altogether, this finding suggests that a child's experience of listening to music is a far more active experience than it initially appears.

Music can also be experienced as a *participatory* activity, in which children are engaged in the experience of creating the music themselves; this might take the form of learning a musical instrument or making up songs and rhymes in musical play (Marsh & Young, 2006). Yet from a young age, children experience music principally as an *interactive,* social medium; for instance, mother-and-baby music classes, dancing and singing with friends, sharing love of a latest pop song or singers on the television. Music involves and affords emotional and communicative engagement with the other people (Cross, 2001, 2009; Cross & Woodruff, 2009; Huron, 2001; Ruud, 2008). Whether a child listens to music or plays or interacts with others through music, each of these three modes of experiencing music, which in practice inevitably overlap, has profound influences for children's development.

Research also suggests that engagement with music may have a positive effect on children's skills and capacities outside of the musical context. This is generally referred to as a 'transfer of skills' or the 'transfer effect', in which certain capacities practiced and acquired in one domain can influence or improve skills in a completely different domain (Hallam, 2010).

This chapter explores, through case study and research from our multiple disciplines, how three identified modes of musical engagement—music *listening*, music *learning*, and musical *interaction* with others—can impact a child's development. We frame this chapter around the three main areas of child development for children aged 5 to 12 years: cognitive, physical, and social-emotional development. The first section will examine research and clinical knowledge concerning the *cognitive* developments associated with music listening, formal instrumental learning, and collective musical interaction in childhood. The next section will discuss research and clinical knowledge of *physical* developments associated with music listening, playing instruments, and music-making with others, while the following section will consider research and clinical knowledge in the areas of *social-emotional* developments and music listening, collective musical interaction, and formal instrumental learning. In each of these sections we consider how and why music affords such developments for children. In the next section, we go on to call for further interdisciplinary methods and collaboration, which we see as lacking in existing research, followed in the final section by a discussion of the conclusions and future directions.

At a time of vast and rapid change in a child's cognitive, physical, social, and emotional development, music can have a profound significance and influence on the care and nurture of an individual. In this chapter, we explore from an interdisciplinary perspective how musical care, in a multitude of modalities, nurtures the quality of the developing child's interactions with the world.

Musical care and the cognitive development of children

Research from music psychology and music education has demonstrated a possible link between listening to music, instrumental learning, and typically developing children's cognitive development (Jaschke et al., 2018; Schlaug et al., 2005). Cognition refers to the range of processes required for us to 'think'; i.e., how we store information and subsequently use that information to guide our behaviour. Cognition fundamentally controls our thoughts, decisions, and actions and is therefore critical for everyday living.

Children develop and acquire cognitive skills through interaction with the world around them (Tudge & Rogoff, 1999). Throughout childhood, children's thought processing changes dramatically, because they are constantly developing cognitive skills such as spatial awareness, memory, verbal skills, and general intelligence, all of which play a role in the way a child behaves, feels, and interacts. Researchers have studied various modes of musical engagement and their relationship with multiple cognitive skills in children:

Spatial ability is the capacity to judge and remember spatial relationships between objects, and the ability to visualize within the mind's eye. Schellenberg and Hallam (2005) found that after listening to pre-recorded music, older children (within our previously defined age bracket) benefit from enhanced spatial abilities. Specifically, when 10- to 11-year-old children listened to familiar pop songs and classical music during spatial reasoning tasks, such as jigsaws and block building, they performed faster and more accurately than children not listening to any music (Schellenberg & Hallam, 2005). It is possible that when listening to music, we tend to think in an abstract manner—imagining movement or imagining watching a performer (Zatorre et al., 2007) and indeed we know that neurons related to movement are activated when we are listening to music (Iacoboni et al., 1999). We suggest that this physical awareness awoken when we are listening to music possibly transfers into enhanced spatial-ability reasoning.

Previous studies demonstrated that listening to music may improve children's performance in *memory tasks*, specifically the ability to store and recall new information. Hallam et al. (2002) report that 10- to 12-year-old children listening to calm pre-recorded music perform better on memory tasks compared with children who listened to arousing or unpleasant music, or children who did not listen to any kind of music at all. This finding may suggest that the effects of listening to music on a child's memory may be related to the emotion the music evokes in the child. We already know that music listening affects our mood and emotions (Juslin & Sloboda, 2011) and that positive mood enables better concentration and therefore possibly a better capacity to store relevant information (Loewenstein & Lerner, 2003). One could speculate that mood-related effects of listening to music might be the underlying reason that music may improve children's working memory. Taken together, these studies on music listening suggest a transfer of skills and capacities that enhance a child's cognitive development: specifically spatial abilities and working memory.

The act of learning to play musical instruments inevitably entails an advanced level of involvement and the memorizing and execution of specific skills and abilities, such as fine motor movement and co-ordination, pattern recognition in sheet-music reading, and the translation of symbols into a physical action. Portowitz et al. (2009) report that learning a musical instrument contributes to better performance in *visual memory* tasks of children aged 5 to 10. Ho et al. (2003) show that children aged 6 to 15 with long-term training on a musical instrument perform better at *verbal memory* tasks than children without any musical training up to a year after receiving instrumental tuition. Indeed, children need to access stored memories of learned skills in order to play music. It is therefore likely that exercising memory skills through learning a musical instrument transfers to a general ability to store and recall information in everyday contexts (Snyder, 2000).

Verbal intelligence is the ability to analyse and problem-solve by using language-based reasoning; it might involve reading, listening to words, conversing, or writing. Moreno et al. (2011) found that children aged 4 to 6 who took part in a four-week music program of computerized pitch, voice, and rhythm perception tasks showed significantly greater improvements in tests of verbal intelligence than children taking part in an art programme. Longer periods of musical instrument training also suggest specific effects on children's auditory pitch discrimination skills in language perception. For example, Habibi et al. (2016) observed that, after 2 years of a music tuition programme, children, aged 6 to 7 at the start of the study enhanced their ability to detect pitch changes in language and showed an accelerated maturity of auditory processing compared with children involved in non-music programmes. Further still, an electroencephalogram (EEG) study demonstrated at the neural level that instrumental music training had a positive impact on 8-year-old children's capacity to detect pitch patterns in language compared to children with no instrumental training (Magne et al., 2006). A large part of verbal intelligence is the auditory processing of language, which is reliant on well-developed listening skills (Smoski et al., 1992). When children play music and learn to play instruments, they are practising detailed *listening skills*—attuning themselves to tonal inflections, rhythmicity, and learning to imitate and interpret what they hear through their own playing (Kraus & Chandrasekaran, 2010). Indeed, Schellenberg and Weiss (2013) found that musical training is correlated with high-ability speech skills, including the perception of intonation and stresses in speech, and phonological perception. Given the results of these few studies, it is possible to suggest that musical training may have the potential to enhance aspects of children's verbal and linguistic intelligence.

Children's *global intelligence quotient* (IQ) has been shown to have a strong positive relationship with musical aptitude and musical training (Swaminathan et al., 2017). Learning to play music involves the practising and simultaneous exercising of a multitude of cognitive functions that are all relevant to a child's intelligence, including focused attention and concentration, memorization, acute listening, fine motor activity, and often the reading of a complex notation system. Indeed, studies have suggested that the duration of learning an instrument for children aged 6 to 11 was correlated with overall greater general intelligence (Schellenberg, 2006).

Taken together, studies on music learning suggest that learning how to play music instigates a transfer of skills and capacities that may enhance a child's cognitive development; from visual and linguistic memory and listening skills through to global intelligence or IQ (see also Schellenberg, 2005).

The opportunity to interact while a child is playing music with others in formal groups such as orchestras, ensembles, and choirs offers a further set of possible outcomes. The act of playing music with other people requires a child to pay attention simultaneously to their own playing and to other people's musical utterances (Cross et al., 2012; Trevarthen & Aitken, 2001). This requirement means that the child has to engage their *visual, motor, and auditory skills* in relation to others in order to stay in time and in tune with others. Four- to 6-year-old children who participated in Kindermusik—interactive group music-making classes with their parents—showed *enhanced spatial memory ability*. Specifically, they showed an improved ability to remember and reproduce sequences of coloured beads, compared to control groups (Bilhartz et al., 1999). Children aged 8 years old who had participated in interactive group music lessons for 6 months were found to have better *reading skills*, compared with children in painting lessons (Moreno, 2009), while 4- to 6-year-old children taking part in computerized music training programmes for 20 days outperformed children taking part in computerized visual art programmes on *verbal intelligence* tests (Moreno et al., 2011). Burnard (2000, 2002) found that following participation in interactive group music-making classes in schools, 5- to 10-year-old children had greater *imaginative thinking* than children who had not had any extra musical input at school. It is important to note that for most of the studies exploring the relationship between participation in a group music activity and cognitive growth in children, no overall gain in intelligence was detected; the effects that were found were specific to the tasks performed and defined areas of cognition (Mehr et al., 2013). However, as previously mentioned, Schellenberg (2006) found that the duration of learning an instrument for children aged 6 to 11 was correlated with overall greater general intelligence.

Music therapy research—primarily through qualitative research and case studies—discusses the specific role of musical interaction and how it may influence children's cognitive skills, such as auditory and linguistic processing, listening skills, memory, and attention (Pavlicevic, 1999; Wheeler, 2005). Music therapy, which in these cases involves active playing, singing, and improvisation between the music therapist and client(s), has been shown to increase the amount of time that children with autism spectrum disorders (ASDs) are able to engage in instances of *joint attention* both in and outside of therapy (Kim et al., 2008; Vaiouli et al., 2015). Music therapists use a variety of musical techniques to engage a child and work towards goals (Bunt et al., 2013; Pavlicevic, 2003). Such techniques could involve encouraging the copying of rhythmic patterns, including variation of rhythmic subdivisions and groupings, which may well enhance the ability to understand mathematical principals such as proportion, patterns, and subdivision, because it calls upon similar cognitive functions (Schlaug et al., 2005). Children may also be encouraged to sing or speak in a regular rhythm, or the therapist may leave spaces in songs for the child to fill in to help stimulate speech. Such techniques that are intended to encourage speech and language have the potential to lead to cognitive gains, because processing of both music and language requires the capacity to segment sounds into smaller perceptual units (Schlaug et al., 2005) in order to enable understanding.

The following vignette, drawn from the clinical music therapy experience of one of the authors', illustrates the case of a boy who had severe speech and language regression due to a seizure-related condition. Interacting, expressing, and practicing skills through long-term, regular music therapy sessions supported his capacity for expression and communication with the people around him.

Francis

This case study concerns a 5-year-old boy with Landau-Kleffner syndrome. Francis had functioned normally up to the age of 5, when he had a sudden period of regression in all language-related areas. He lost all active and passive language, and the ability to talk, make eye contact, and play. He was highly anxious, had a very short concentration span, and was unable to sit still.

Music therapy could support Francis, having lost all of his communication skills, with the building blocks of learning—listening, attention, awareness of and interacting with others, turn taking, and speech. Initially these aims were worked on primarily nonverbally by using just the music and techniques such as sharing a basic beat, copying and then elaborating on rhythmic patterns in turn taking, leaving spaces in the music for the child to finish the phrase, and later adding sounds and then language into these exchanges. Music also allowed him to maintain engagement with someone else despite being very physically active and moving around the room.

At the beginning Francis was interested in playing the drum and cymbal—often very loudly—but clearly with great satisfaction, smiling and moving his body as the therapist accompanied him in the Blues style. Large percussion instruments were positioned around the room so that he could come in and out of playing as he moved, and the joy that he found in this experience of shared meaning in making music, his smiles and laughter and sense of fun revealing his personality, was tangible. Friday mornings after his music therapy session were the one time in the week that Francis would go willingly into his mainstream school, where he was very much on the periphery of all learning, unable to engage and highly anxious. It was as though with some confidence restored, he had been fortified by the satisfaction of meaningful connection with others and himself, through the music.

As Francis began to settle into sessions, and become less jumpy, the therapist brought a violin and cello for him to experiment with. His progress in settling down and briefly being able to focus, and use some words again, was also a result of medication stopping the epileptic activity, allowing new neural pathways to be formed, and relearning to begin.

In addition to the cognitive benefits that enhanced his communication skills, music therapy also offered Francis an expressive outlet. Towards the end of his year of music therapy he regularly engaged with focus and intention, played the violin and cello, and improvised in a trio with the therapist and his mother.

Such cognition- and language-related music therapy case studies are many (Pavlicevic, 1999) and often relate to language rebuilding, in the case of adult stroke patients (Ansdell, 1995), or *language acquisition* for young children with autism (Gold et al., 2006). The majority of large-scale quantitative research studies that focus on specific aspects of cognition are inevitably from the music psychology and education disciplines. Drawing together the fields of music psychology, music education research, and music therapy, a focus on the potential benefits of cognitive development within music therapy sessions with non-typically developing child populations would be a particularly useful future collaboration that could help to highlight what aspects of music therapy work can best support children with cognitive challenges.

These modes of musical engagement—listening, learning, or interacting with others—potentially offer opportunities for children to develop multiple cognitive processes (Kersten, 2015; Schellenberg & Weiss, 2013). Combined, the studies from music psychology, music education, and music therapy suggest that engaging with musical care could support a wide range of a child's developing cognitive processes; from spatial visualization and memory to verbal processing, listening, and language skills. Music in many modalities nurtures multiple areas of cognitive development across the span of middle childhood.

Musical care for physiological functioning and physical development of children

Dancing, moving, tapping, and nodding—engaging with music draws out an instinctive motor response that is evident from an early age (Kirschner & Tomasello, 2009), as was seen in the Musical care in infancy chapter. Children gradually develop strength, speed, sensory processes, and coordination throughout childhood. The physical development of children aged 5 to 12 encompasses a wide range of physical ability. Most 5-year-olds have not yet developed fine motor control, so struggle with the coordination of smaller, detailed movements such as writing, whereas an 11-year-old has further developed fine motor skills and is capable of fine-detailed and nuanced movements (Carlson et al., 2013; Mussen & Conger, 1956). Physical development activities and experiences are a crucial part of a child's care and autonomy in general daily life.

Playing music inevitably involves the intricate coordination of a series of fine motor movements—the use of small muscles in the hands, fingers, and wrists in synchronization with the eyes—and gross motor skills—larger limb and whole-body movements such as jumping and walking (Schlaug et al., 2005). Yet research studies and observations indicate that while listening to and learning and interacting through music, not only can children experience *physical* change in the way they move, use, and coordinate their body's actions, but also music can influence their bodies' *physiological* functioning—their experience and perception of physical sensation.

Research suggests that listening to music can *reduce pain* for children and infants in the NICU, as is described in the Musical care in infancy chapter. Painful traumatic experiences in a child's early life can shape and inform how they respond to stimuli in later life (Young, 2005). Reducing a child's distress and experience of physical pain can therefore reduce the chance of long-lasting negative consequences. Bradt (2010) and Miladinia et al. (2016) found that playing pre-recorded music to children during and after operations reduced 8- to 18-year-old children's experience of pain, compared with those who did not listen to any music. The age of the children did not impact the effectiveness in reducing pain, so the results remain true for younger children. Nguyen et al. (2010) found that 7- to 12-year-old children listening to pre-recorded music felt *less anxious* undergoing operations than children not listening to music. This response was likely because listening to music can induce a positive mood in children, which may result in lower anxiety. Moreover, Uggla et al. (2016) showed that listening to live performed music *lowered the heart rate* and anxiety levels of children aged 6 to 18 in a paediatric oncology unit before operations, an effect that could be attributed to the music distracting the child from the intensity of the pain (Aitken et al., 2002; Kwekkeboom, 2003). The experience of pain is influenced by the psychological and emotional processes of every individual; it is a partially subjective sensory process (Koyama et al., 2005). It has been shown that stress levels, anxiety, and therefore a negative mood worsen a person's experience of pain (Cassady et al., 2004; Isen & Labroo, 2003). However, we also know that listening to preferred music positively changes children's mood (Schellenberg & Hallam, 2005), inducing a release of neurochemicals, such as the neurotransmitter dopamine, which inhibits the release of the body's stress hormone cortisol (Dunlop & Nemeroff, 2007) and promotes a relaxation effect. Though listening to music does not remove the source of pain, the mood modulating effect of listening to pre-recorded or live music is a viable reason for children to experience a reduction in their perception of pain.

Further studies from music education extend knowledge regarding the physiological effects of musical care by specifically examining the effect of children's music-making on the release of the hormone cortisol (higher levels of which contribute to feelings of *stress*; Brown et al., 2017) show that preschool-aged children participating in taught group music classes have lower levels of cortisol immediately after music classes and in the long term, compared with children taking dance or visual arts classes. Lindblad et al. (2007) show similar outcomes compared with children not participating in any extracurricular activities. We suggest that both listening to and physically playing music with others nurtures children at a physiological level.

Music can nurture children at a basic physical level. Children experience vast changes in the way they move and use their bodies, and coordinate their bodies' actions between the ages of 5 and 12. Children require exercise and movement activities to build strength and muscle tone and to practice coordination for normal physical development. Learning to play instruments exercises *fine motor skill*, while the natural impulse to move and dance to music encourages *gross motor movements* made with our limbs or entire bodies. Observational studies from music education research note 4- to 6-year-old children's ability to throw, catch, jump, skip, and leap improved when they participated in music workshops focused on teaching rhythm (Beisman, 1967; Derri et al., 2001). Brown et al. (1981) reported that a combined music and physical education programme improved 4- to 6-year-old children's gross motor skills more than a movement-only programme. Learning a musical instrument inevitably gets a child regularly practising fine motor coordination and dexterity for performing complex patterns (Costa-Giomi, 2005; Schlaug et al., 2005). Indeed, evidence suggests that children of all ages who learn to play a musical instrument have better fine motor skills than children who are not musically trained (Norton et al., 2005; Schlaug et al., 2005). Music training or extensive exposure to music throughout childhood has been shown to help older children, aged 10 to 14 years, develop the ability to synchronize their own physical movements. Such children are more accurate at moving in synchrony with a constant beat and maintaining a regular beat than children who have little exposure to music (Janzen et al., 2014). These studies suggest that learning a musical instrument trains a child's motor system specifically with regard to timed movements.

The ability to control and *synchronize movements in time* is an important skill for children to develop that relies on the interaction between physical and perceptual skill (Phillips-Silver & Keller, 2012). The ability to control the *timing* of movements and gestures has implications for the performance of everyday motoric tasks, like getting onto an escalator, or even being able to successfully communicate and socially interact with gestures (Cassell et al., 1994; Goldin-Meadow, 1999). Indeed, interactive music therapy has been shown to improve autistic children's motor skills, such as copying movements when engaging in normal social exchanges and conversations (Hardy & LaGasse, 2013). Two studies from music psychology research show that children more accurately time their drumming movements when playing with a social partner rather than with an auditory-only drumbeat (Ilari et al., 2018; Kirschner & Tomasello, 2009). Such physical outcomes for non-typically developing children are prevalent within music therapy research and literature. For instance, Rickson (2006) suggests that facilitated interactive music-making may improve the motor impulsivity of older children and adolescents (11- to 15-year-olds) with attention deficit hyperactivity disorder (ADHD); participants in interactive music therapy sessions were more able to synchronize their playing accurately with another person's beat in comparison with those not taking part in interactive music therapy sessions.

Taken together, this research suggests that playing together with another person (the socially interactive context) enables children to accurately synchronize their motor movements, more than playing alone while following a computerized external beat. When playing music with another person, a child is given visual as well as auditory clues for synchronizing accurately; children also learn to attend and respond to microphysical signals in their partners' gestures that help them to adapt towards and understand their partners' intentions (Lively et al., 1993). The social musical context provides children with more stimuli for learning how to 'read' another person's intentions and therefore synchronize their movements with them. Music psychology research indicates that this exercise leads to enhanced empathy; a key component in forming relationships and getting on with others in childhood and adult life (Rabinowitch et al., 2013; Rabinowitch & Meltzoff, 2017b). Such research outcomes help to uncover the relationship between children's physical skills and social-emotional skills; the latter are described in the next section of this chapter.

The specifically interactive setting of music making seems to promote *physical strength and flexibility* outcomes for children suffering from physically limiting conditions. Wu et al. (2008) observed that children with cerebral palsy benefit from physically stretching while playing music in therapy sessions and show an increase in physical strength. Wu et al. also report that children who had engaged in interactive musical activities during sessions, i.e., using percussion, singing, and dancing, as well as acupuncture treatment, benefited from greater freedom of physical movement and flexibility than children who received only acupuncture treatment. Music therapists working with children with a physical disability often encourage movement and stretching through gradually increasing the distance children have to reach towards instruments in order to play (Wigram, 2004). The enjoyment of the activity may motivate children to try harder and therefore see greater improvements in physical ability than undergoing physical exercises without music.

Music therapists can use music to encourage physical exercise and movement, such as stretching, reaching, walking, jumping, clapping, and gripping (Paul & Ramsey, 2000). Drawn from the clinical experience of one of the authors, the following vignette illustrates how music plays a vital role in the physical care of a girl with severe developmental delay due to a genetic condition. Practicing and using songs to accompany everyday tasks nurtures her capacity for understanding, independence in daily life, and physical expression.

Martha

Martha is a 5-year-old girl with a rare genetic syndrome, microcephaly, and significant developmental delay. Martha attends a small group for preschool children and their parents/carers at a music therapy centre. The weekly 30-minute sessions are a mixture of activities that offer a range of experiences. Framing the session with a familiar hello song and a goodbye song, the therapist chooses from a range of possible activities. These include listening or moving to rhyme and action songs; copying movements, and/or placing sounds/words at the end of phrases; offering small percussion instruments for the children to choose and play together in free improvisation, supported and reflected in the music by the therapist at the piano; offering each child the chance to play in a 'drum' song or 'bell' song at a particular place in the music, and so allowing them the anticipation and satisfaction of ending the phrase, for example. Thus, each child has the chance to hear themselves together with others or by themselves. They have the opportunity to experiment with different instruments and sounds, to be part of familiar musical structures, and to create their own music.

Martha's mother used songs and activities from the sessions to help life at home. For instance, she changed words in a stretching song to make them fit into a 'getting-your vest-off' song. When asked about the benefits of music therapy she noted in particular how it had helped with physical challenges, saying, 'Music and what we've learnt through it has been a real boost to Martha. We have seen how music makes words and concepts more memorable and using this at home has made an enormous difference to daily routines, not just play. It has made things like dressing, physio, and toileting more understandable and fun, and is definitely a big player in Martha's progress with them.'

Musical care can transform the daily experiences of children with physical disabilities—building strength and providing motivation to help perform daily living skills. When that kind of care is combined with research from music psychology and music education, we are given a broader picture of how music nurtures a child's physical development. There is a range of research, particularly from music therapy and music psychology, that looks at children affected by illness or developmental conditions. There is less research in this area from the world of music education beyond the enhanced fine motor skills of children learning instruments. Existing research focuses on the use of music as a tool that nurtures and supports children with a physical disability or illness: i.e., music to reduce pain in operations, to facilitate stretching for children with physically limiting conditions, or to improve impulsivity in children with ADHD. This use produces a new set of questions; if music 'works' for these vulnerable populations of children, will it also 'work' for typically developing child populations to extend their existing capabilities?

Music research in the area of physical development stresses the unequivocal functionality of music in caring for children. Whether for listening, learning to play, or interacting with others, each mode of musical engagement offers opportunities for children's physiological functioning and physical development to be nurtured throughout their childhood.

Musical care and the social-emotional development of children

A child's emotional development involves both intra- and interpersonal processes; throughout childhood, children develop the ability to identify, understand, and regulate their own emotions, but also recognize and respond to the emotional states of others (Denham, 1998). A child's emotional development is strongly linked to their functioning in relation to others (Holmes, 1993), which is partly why social development and emotional development are often grouped together. Social and emotional growth is necessary for children to be able to develop basic life skills and capacities such as empathy, co-operation, self-control, confidence, adaptability, and attention (Phillips & Shonkoff, 2000). These capacities and skills help children become competent in managing emotional responses to life experiences, to negotiate complex social interactions, and to participate effectively in relationships and group activities in order to be able to access and benefit from social support networks crucial for healthy development and functioning.

By the age of 7, children have been shown to have strong learned music-emotion associations (Gregory et al., 1996). Hallam et al. (2002) found that listening to music can not only change a child's mood, but can also increase their helpful behaviours towards others, possibly because of the connection found between mood and prosocial behaviour (Brief & Motowidlo, 1986; George, 1991). Therefore, children who listen to pieces of music or songs that make them feel more positive are more likely to be socially attentive and helpful.

When children engage in music through learning an instrument or singing, there are further interpersonal gains. In order to relate to another person and behave in an emotionally appropriate way towards them, children gradually develop the ability to predict or 'read' the emotions of other people and adapt their behaviour accordingly (Moore, 2017). Schellenberg and Mankarious (2012) showed that children who were musically trained were more able to identify emotions in others—an indicator of *empathic capacity*. Because music learning can lead to such gains in social-emotional skills, this ability may be a contributing factor in the raised *self-esteem* and *confidence* of children who are musically trained. As noted in a study by Costa-Giomi (2004), children who had engaged in three years of piano tuition were found to have higher ratings of self-esteem than children who had not received any formal music instruction. Gaining a skill that others do not necessarily have is a boost to a child's self-comparison with peers. Children compare their own social standing and intellectual and artistic abilities with those of others from a young age (Festinger, 1954). It is possible that children who have nurtured a 'talent' have an improved self-perception and self-identity compared with their peers. Further studies are needed in order to establish whether this effect is music-specific or general in nature and whether the musical training is the cause for these effects, or whether those with better self-perception and self-identity are more likely to engage in music learning (see Butkovic et al., 2015; Corrigall et al., 2013; Corrigall & Schellenberg, 2015; Mosing et al., 2016; Swaminathan et al., 2017; Theorell et al., 2015).

Engagement with music in a socially interactive setting seems to offer an array of social-emotional outcomes for children. A therapeutic music context is particularly beneficial for the *emotional regulation* and *emotional stability* of children with ASD (Carpente, 2016) and for children experiencing traumatic circumstances (Baker & Jones, 2006; Porter et al., 2017). Music psychology studies suggest that music interaction and song writing in groups reduce childhood depression and anxiety for children with separated families (DeLucia-Waack & Gellman, 2007; Hilliard, 2001), while music therapy studies also note anxiety reduction as a key outcome of interactive music-making in groups of children with learning disabilities and children admitted to hospital (Dykens et al., 2005; Hooper & Lindsay, 1990). Having an outlet for emotional self-expression through engagement with verbal or nonverbal creativity is related to positive emotional health and self-confidence (Berry & Pennebaker, 1993).

Several studies have shown that musical interaction can also nurture a child's capacity for *empathy* and *prosociality*. Rabinowitch et al. (2013) found that long-term participation in group music-making, focused on musical activities involving adaptation and attentiveness to others, can enhance 8- to 11-year-old children's capacity for empathy. Good & Russo (2016) found that older children displayed more prosocial and co-operative behaviours after taking part in a short-term music groups involving adaptation activities, compared to children who did not take part. Similarly, Kirschner & Tomasello (2010) found that 4-year-olds showed more prosocial behaviours after taking part in a one-off music session with musical activities focused on collaborative group activities and stories. The musical intervention in each of these three studies focused on music activities that encouraged synchrony, imitation, and joint attention among the participating children. Through experiencing these activities during the music program, children were practising capacities of attending and anticipating the intentions and actions of others. The findings suggest that these capacities were then transferred outside of the music context. After comparison of the music group also with children participating in other, non-musical groups, such as play, drama, arts, or sports, it seems that musical interaction may afford a unique quality of interaction, which may contribute to more positive emotional and social behaviours in children.

Further research suggests that collaborative participation in music activities strengthens and builds *social bonds*. An important feature that distinguishes musical interactions from most other social interactions is the experience of shared rhythm (Bispham, 2006; Merker, 2000). It is possible that this focus on synchrony and shared rhythm is what contributes to enhanced feelings of social bonding when children take part in music activities, compared with other types of social interaction. Several studies have shown how children help (Cirelly et al., 2014; Tuncgenc & Cohen, 2018), cooperate (Rabinowitch & Melztoff, 2017a, 2017b) and bond better (Rabinowitch & Knafo-Noam, 2015; Tuncgenc & Cohen, 2016) following an "experience of being in synchrony with another child or adult". Indeed, this innate instinct to synchronize with others may have evolved specifically *because* synchrony is a mechanism that may help us work together and bond more effectively (Kirschner & Tomasello, 2009; Turino, 2008).

Studies taking place in educational settings found enhanced social integration and relationships between primary-aged children who actively take part in extracurricular group music activities (Hallam, 2010; Pitts, 2007; Spychiger et al., 1993; Sward, 1989). Gooding (2011) and Burnard (2002) note that taking part in musical improvisation groups can lead to significant improvements in *empathic social engagement* among young school children, particularly for those identified as having social deficits.

Part of being able to socially engage with others is the ability to share directed attention, such as to jointly focus on a task with another child or adult. Several studies of music therapy found that improvisational music therapy sessions improved the number of *sustained joint attention* behaviours for children with ASD, compared with play therapy (Kim et al., 2008; LaGasse, 2017; Vaiouli et al., 2015). Music therapists encourage joint attention by using techniques that capture a child's attention: for example, copying their rhythms or tonal phrases, shifting between leading or following in the music, or providing varied musical experiences by shifting the child from a rigid musical beat to an accelerando, or encouraging the child to fill in the last word in each line of a favourite nursery rhyme (Baker & Wigram, 2005; Tomaino, 2012). The flexible use of these techniques aims to maintain a sustained communicative connection with the child. Certainly, a review of music therapy research notes that the varied modes of musical interaction in sessions improve the *communication skills* of children with ASD: specifically, eye contact, eye gaze, and turn taking (Gold et al., 2006). Such musical interaction not only increases children's eye contact with the therapist within sessions, but is also said to transfer out of the session; children with ASD showed an improved ability and willingness to focus on people's faces following music therapy interventions (Vaiouli et al., 2015), a characteristic challenge for children with ASD. Indeed, playing music with others necessitates a variety of looking, listening, adapting, and attending behaviours. Playing music together is a profoundly communicative act, drawing upon many of the same capacities and skills needed for everyday communication and socialization. It is therefore natural that research studies see marked social-emotional improvements among children who participate in flexible, interactive musical activities, like music therapy, as illustrated in the following vignette from one of the author's clinical music therapy work.

Fatima

This case study describes one of two siblings (twins) who were adopted at 7 years old. They were part of a large family and had experienced serious neglect for the first 4.5 years of life. They were then placed in foster care for 2 years and then adopted. Both girls attended mainstream school and showed different degrees of learning difficulties and challenging behaviours, such as extreme anger tantrums and violent outbursts, high anxiety, and self-harming.

In sessions, Fatima's speech was difficult to understand, and she would move around the music room flitting from one instrument to the next, making fleeting eye contact with the therapist and unable to settle at anything. It felt very muddled, and hard to make any sort of connection with her. Beginning and ending the sessions was particularly hard; she was very reluctant to come in at the start; it was then impossible to get her to leave when it was time to finish. As she got used to the situation, she began to allow herself at times to be drawn into the music: for instance, coming to sit by the therapist at the piano during the session-opening 'hello' song, holding her gaze and focus, as the music provided familiarity, a regular pulse and rhythmic impetus that allowed Fatima to organize and calm herself internally and then respond in the music: for example, by playing the keys at the top of the piano. She often wanted to play hide-and-seek, and the therapist would use musical techniques to heighten the suspense as she looked for Fatima, and celebrate finding her, over and over again. There was a period of the therapy in which dad also joined in, with Fatima, who often pretended to be a baby, being cradled in his arms and exchanging nonverbal sounds and expressions. She would then leap back into symbolic play, regularly being the strict teacher in the classroom who wouldn't let anyone in the room do any 'playing' of any kind. At times of heightened anxiety—for example, when going to visit her foster family—she had a desperate need to control sessions, bringing many frustrated and difficult feelings to the room. This atmosphere made it hard to connect with her through any kind of play, be it musical, early, or symbolic. The therapist would reflect musically, also using words, on Fatima's behaviour in sessions, hoping to support Fatima to begin to become more self-aware.

These themes show Fatima experimenting with expressing and regulating her emotions; working to engage and sustain motivation in musical interaction; and exploring relating to others, whether through interactions developmentally appropriate for a much younger child, giving her the chance to compensate for earlier deficits by reworking early patterns of interaction, or in roles that made her feel in control when she was less able to be spontaneous. Fatima's dad noted how music therapy sessions made Fatima 'feel more comfortable in her own skin'. They also played a role in helping her to gradually settle at school and begin to learn and cope in that environment.

The connection between music and emotion has been researched and written about widely within music psychology and music therapy disciplines (Bunt & Pavlicevic, 2001; Juslin & Sloboda, 2011) and will also be discussed in the next chapter on Musical care in adolescence). There is a clear relationship between music and emotion that many of us can relate to and therefore do not question. However, the previously mentioned studies explored delve further to attribute certain musical components with specific social-emotional outcomes: for example, the relationship between synchrony and empathy (Rabinowitch et al., 2013). Equally, the need for a child's emotional world to be nurtured and cared for is implicit in contemporary psychological thought (Perry, 2020), so music's role in nurturing a child's social-emotional growth is accepted. Therefore, there is a need for further studies that explore *how* children's emotional development can be musically nurtured: what qualities of music, what styles and modes of interaction, and for how long?

The aforementioned research explored features a variety of approaches to engaging children in music; however, the most common approach in investigating music and social-emotional development is through interactive music groups, including music therapy client-therapist dyads. There is less child-focused research on the social-emotional implications of music listening and learning. The social element is a key player in children's emotional development. The outcomes of musical care for the emotional development of a child range from the intrapersonal (self-esteem, confidence, emotional regulation) through to the interpersonal (empathy, social bonding, communication skills).

Children's social and emotional development rapidly changes during middle childhood and many studies suggest that early experiences, relationships, and interactions influence and shape a person's personality (Belski et al., 1991; Caspi & Shiner, 2006). Musical care, in a multitude of modalities, has the potential to nurture empathic capacities, prosocial behaviours and communication skills in the developing child.

A call for interdisciplinary methods and collaboration

Our overview of research knowledge could have easily fallen into findings from the separate disciplines of music psychology, music education, music and health, and music therapy. Yet despite the fact that listening, learning, and interacting often co-occur, our categorizations by such musical mode still did not entirely avoid these disciplinary separations. Many of the studies depicted in the music listening sections are derived from the music psychology literature; much of the music learning literature concerns instrumental tuition from the music education field; and much of the music interaction literature is drawn from music therapy research. Though there is some overlap, each discipline could benefit from expanding its research into other modes of musical engagement. Furthermore, music therapy research and literature naturally focus on non-typically developing children. In contrast, it is notable that other fields of music research, specifically music psychology and education, for the most part, do not explore the effects of music on children with additional needs.

In general, music psychology research tends to be quantitative in nature, whereas music therapy research tends to be qualitative. Research in music education contexts can bridge both methodologies; however, researchers do not tend to address the ancillary effects of music. Both quantitative and qualitative research methodologies, and especially their combination, could provide an even richer platform for exploring questions regarding the benefits of musical engagement on children's development. There is therefore a need to develop interdisciplinary research methods that appropriately and systematically capture the changes observed in children involved in musical interventions, from both quantitative and qualitative vantage points. The largest body of evidence for the efficacy of music therapy is case-study-based, or report-based and is generated from within the music therapy profession (Darnley-Smith & Patey, 2003; Pavlicevic, 1999; Robarts, 2006). There has been an effort in recent years to conduct systematic studies by using replicable methods, including control groups and standardized outcome measures (Geretsegger et al., 2012; Kim et al., 2008; Kim et al., 2009; Spiro & Himberg, 2016); yet the conflict between the necessarily flexible music therapy aims, which emerge spontaneously with the child's changing needs (Bunt et al., 2013; Darnley-Smith & Patey, 2003; Odell, 1988; Oldfield, 2006), compared with the necessary rigidity of research aims, has resulted in few attempts to conduct such research and inconclusive results in some instances (Aydin & Sahiner, 2017; Bieleninik et al., 2017; Lim & Draper, 2011). There is therefore a need for more interdisciplinary collaboration to enable cross-methodological experimental designs that can capture the full breadth of musical engagement in music therapy research.

An additional issue is the duration of the music 'intervention' employed in each study. The positive outcomes of musical care that potentially transfer to a child's daily life can be long and short term, yet the length of research studies concerning children and music is generally short term; several studies examined benefits after a single session (Kirschner & Tomasello, 2010); some involved a short succession of sessions lasting 6 to 8 weeks (Mehr et al., 2016; Moreno et al., 2011) and longer studies lasted 1 school year (Rabinowitch et al., 2013 ; Schellenberg & Mankarious, 2012). Only rarely does a study examine longer periods of time, such as 3 years (Ilari et al., 2018). Considering that music is something that children engage with throughout their childhood and beyond, it is notable that so few studies are longitudinal in nature. Studies that follow up with participants post intervention to test for retention effects are especially scarce.

Finally, in order to establish a *causal* role of long-term musical interventions in the modulation of any behaviour or cognitive, emotional, or social capacity, many researchers may highlight the importance of randomization in the experimental design as far as practically possible within clinical and educational settings. For instance, in many studies the child participants themselves often elect whether to participate or not in the musical activities. Such non-randomized designs can be criticized in that the choice to participate could play a role in any observed behavioural outcomes rather than the music itself, so efforts should be made to rule out this possibility and strengthen data findings (Habibi et al., 2014). Conversely, real-world applicability is an important part of conducting research. As randomized controlled trials are expensive and complex to conduct, research rigor has to balance with practicality and applicability.

The observations that we have described highlight the potential knowledge that can be gained by further interdisciplinary collaboration. Music is multimodal, is multifaceted, and offers benefits for children in a multitude of domains; research should reflect all this. Music psychologists, educators, and therapists can work together to find ways of researching real-world music. The availability of new technologies combined with collaborative multidisciplinary research design has the potential to further illuminate the dynamics and potentials of children's engagement with music. Indeed, the limits of music research should not be governed by narrowly defined professional disciplines, but by the pervasive nature of music itself.

Conclusions and future directions

Exploration of existing research from a variety of disciplines—music psychology, music therapy, and music education—has given us a holistic view of *how* and *why* music nurtures a child's development. Drawing together these perspectives, research and findings have helped to broaden our understanding of how different modalities—listening, learning, and interacting—of music nurture a child's cognitive, physical, and social-emotional development.

The research-based cognitive outcomes of musical care for children explored in this chapter range from improved spatial abilities and IQ to enhanced memory and verbal intelligence. However, existing studies are small scale and few in number, and the effect sizes are small. Indeed, Sala & Gobet (2017) note that the results of such studies are therefore unreliable. Further research is required in order to be able to make any wider claims about music's care for a child's cognitive development.

Musical care for a child's physical development has more easily measurable effects; outcomes from the research explored range from *physiological* outcomes, such as pain reduction, relaxation, and reduced secretion of the stress hormone cortisol, to *physical* outcomes, such as improved gross and fine motor skills, temporal coordination, strength, and greater ability to synchronize with others.

Social-emotional outcomes of musical care for children are well evidenced across the disciplines. Possible gains range from changes in intrapersonal capacities such as self-esteem, confidence, emotional regulation, and stability to changes in interpersonal capacities including empathy, social relationships and bonding, shared attention, and communication skills. Despite the breadth of research describing gains in these areas, it is important to emphasize that it is not necessarily music *per se* that carries a unique power, but it is *how* a child engages musically that may ultimately lead to beneficial developments. Much music therapy literature emphasizes the *ways in which* musical care is employed. As researchers and clinicians, we feel the aim of future music and child-focused research is not only to expand academic knowledge, but also to influence *how* music is used in a child's daily life to nurture cognitive, physical, and social-emotional change and growth.

Children's cognitive, physical, social, and emotional growth develop at a rapid rate between chlldren's ages of 5 and 12 (Papalia et al., 2007; Piaget & Inhelder, 2008; Shaffer, 2013). Childhood experiences have an undeniable impact on a person's adult relationships, choices, personality, and careers (Belski et al., 1991; Caspi & Shiner, 2007), so ensuring that a child has all the necessary skills to take into adult life is an important responsibility. Musical care in childhood simultaneously influences the quality of a child's multiple interactions with the world around them. Musical care is therefore one way to nurture children's cognitive, physical, and social-emotional capacities and help ready them to enter into the next stage of life.

References

Aitken, J. C., Wilson, S., Coury, D., & Moursi, A. M. (2002). The effect of music distraction on pain, anxiety and behavior in pediatric dental patients. *Pediatric Dentistry, 24*(2), 114–118.

Ansdell, G. (1995). *Music for life: Aspects of creative music therapy with adult clients* (Vol. 1). Jessica Kingsley Publishers.

Aydin, D., & Sahiner, N. C. (2017). Effects of music therapy and distraction cards on pain relief during phlebotomy in children. *Applied Nursing Research, 33*, 164–168.

Baker, F., & Wigram, T. (2005). *Songwriting: Methods, techniques and clinical applications for music therapy clinicians, educators and students.* Jessica Kingsley Publishers.

Baker, F., & Jones, C. (2006). The effect of music therapy services on classroom behaviours of newly arrived refugee students in Australia—A pilot study. *Emotional and Behavioural Difficulties, 11*(4), 249–260.

Beisman, G. L. (1967). Effect of rhythmic accompaniment upon learning of fundamental motor skills. *Research Quarterly: American Association for Health, Physical Education and Recreation, 38*(2), 172–176.

Belsky, J., Steinberg, L., & Draper, P. (1991). Childhood experience, interpersonal development, and reproductive strategy: An evolutionary theory of socialization. *Child Development, 62*(4), 647–670.

Bergeson, T. R., & Trehub, S. E. (2007). Signature tunes in mothers' speech to infants. *Infant Behavior and Development, 30*(4), 648–654.

Berry, D. S., & Pennebaker, J. W. (1993). Nonverbal and verbal emotional expression and health. *Psychotherapy and Psychosomatics, 59*(1), 11–19.

Bieleninik, Ł., Geretsegger, M., Mössler, K., Assmus, J., Thompson, G., Gattino, G., & Muratori, F. (2017). Effects of improvisational music therapy vs enhanced standard care on symptom severity among children with autism spectrum disorder: The TIME-A randomized clinical trial. *JAMA, 318*(6), 525–535.

Bilhartz, T. D., Bruhn, R. A., & Olson, J. E. (1999). The effect of early music training on child cognitive development. *Journal of Applied Developmental Psychology, 20*(4), 615–636.

Bispham, J. (2006). Rhythm in music: What is it? Who has it? And why? *Music Perception: An Interdisciplinary Journal, 24*(2), 125–134.

Bradt, J. (2010). The effects of music entrainment on postoperative pain perception in pediatric patients. *Music and Medicine, 2*(3), 150–157.

Brief, A. P., & Motowidlo, S. J. (1986). Prosocial organizational behaviors. *Academy of Management Review, 11*(4), 710–725.

Brown, E. D., Garnett, M. L., Anderson, K. E., & Laurenceau, J. P. (2017). Can the arts get under the skin? Arts and cortisol for economically disadvantaged children. *Child Development, 88*(4), 1368–1381.

Brown, J., Sherrill, C., & Gench, B. (1981). Effects on an integrated physical education /music program in changing early childhood perceptual—motor performance. *Perceptual and Motor Skills, 53,* 51–154.

Bunt, L., & Pavlicevic, M. (2001). *Music and emotion: Perspectives from music therapy.* In P. N. Juslin & J. A. Sloboda (Eds.), *Music and emotion: Theory and research* (pp. 181–201). Oxford University Press.

Bunt, L., Hoskyns, S., & Swami, S. (2013). *The handbook of music therapy.* Routledge.

Burke, H. M., Davis, M. C., Otte, C., & Mohr, D. C. (2005). Depression and cortisol responses to psychological stress: A meta-analysis. *Psychoneuroendocrinology, 30*(9), 846–856.

Burnard, P. (2000). How children ascribe meaning to improvisation and composition: Rethinking pedagogy in music education. *Music Education Research, 2*(1), 7–23.

Burnard, P. (2002). Investigating children's meaning-making and the emergence of musical interaction in group improvisation. *British Journal of Music Education, 19*(2), 157–172.

Butkovic, A., Ullén, F., & Mosing, M. A. (2015). Personality related traits as predictors of music practice: Underlying environmental and genetic influences. *Personality and Individual Differences, 74,* 133–138.

Carlson, A. G., Rowe, E., & Curby, T. W. (2013). Disentangling fine motor skills' relations to academic achievement: The relative contributions of visual-spatial integration and visual-motor coordination. *The Journal of Genetic Psychology, 174*(5), 514–533.

Carpente, J. A. (2016). Investigating the effectiveness of a developmental, individual difference, relationship-based (DIR) improvisational music therapy program on social communication for children with autism spectrum disorder. *Music Therapy Perspectives, 35*(2), 160–174.

Caspi, A., & Shiner, R. L. (2006). *Personality Development.* In N. Eisenberg, W. Damon, & R. M. Lerner (Eds.), *Handbook of child psychology: Social, emotional, and personality development* (pp. 300–365). John Wiley & Sons, Inc.

Cassady, J. C., Mohammed, A., & Mathieu, L. (2004). Cross-cultural differences in test perceptions: Women in Kuwait and the United States. *Journal of Cross-Cultural Psychology, 35*(6), 713–718.

Cassell, J., Pelachaud, C., Badler, N., Steedman, M., Achorn, B., Becket, T., ... & Stone, M. (1994). *Animated conversation: Rule-based generation of facial expression, gesture & spoken intonation for multiple conversational agents.* [Paper presentation]. Proceedings of the 21st Annual Conference on Computer Graphics and Interactive Techniques, New York, USA.

Cirelli, L. K., Einarson, K. M., & Trainor, L. J. (2014). Interpersonal synchrony increases prosocial behavior in infants. *Developmental Science, 17*(6), 1003–1011.

Corrigall, K. A., Schellenberg, E. G., & Misura, N. M. (2013). Music training, cognition, and personality. *Frontiers in Psychology, 4,* 1–10. https://doi.org/10.3389/fpsyg.2013.00222.

Corrigall, K. A., & Schellenberg, E. G. (2015). Predicting who takes music lessons: Parent and child characteristics. *Frontiers in Psychology, 6,* 1–8. https://doi.org/10.3389/fpsyg.2015.00282.

Costa-Giomi, E. (2004). Effects of three years of piano instruction on children's academic achievement, school performance and self-esteem. *Psychology of Music, 32*(2), 139–152.

Costa-Giomi, E. (2005). Does music instruction improve fine motor abilities? *Annals of the New York Academy of Sciences, 1060*(1), 262–264.

Cross, I. (2001). Music, mind and evolution. *Psychology of Music, 29*(1), 95–102.

Cross, I. (2009). The evolutionary nature of musical meaning. *Musicae Scientiae, 13*(2 suppl), 179–200.

Cross, I., & Woodruff, G. E. (2009). Music as a communicative medium. *The Prehistory of Language, 1*, 113–144.

Cross, I., Laurence, F., & Rabinowitch, T.-C. (2012). Empathy and creativity in group musical practices: Towards a concept of empathic creativity. In McPherson, G. E. & Welch, G. F. (Eds.), *The Oxford handbook of music education* (Vol, 2), (pp. 337–358). Oxford University Press.

Darnley-Smith, R., & Patey, H. M. (2003). *Music therapy*. Sage.

DeLucia-Waack, J. L., & Gellman, R. A. (2007). The efficacy of using music in children of divorce groups: Impact on anxiety, depression, and irrational beliefs about divorce. *Group Dynamics: Theory, Research, and Practice, 11*(4), 272.

Denham, S. A. (1998). *Emotional development in young children*. Guilford Press.

Derri, V., Tsapakidou, A., Zachopoulou, E., & Kioumourtzoglou, E. (2001). Effect of a music and movement programme on development of locomotor skills by children 4 to 6 years of age. *European Journal of Physical Education, 6*(1), 16–25.

Dunlop, B. W., & Nemeroff, C. B. (2007). The role of dopamine in the pathophysiology of depression. *Archives of General Psychiatry, 64*(3), 327–337.

Dykens, E. M., Rosner, B. A., Ly, T., & Sagun, J. (2005). Music and anxiety in Williams syndrome: A harmonious or discordant relationship? *American Journal on Mental Retardation, 110*(5), 346–358.

Fernald, A., Taeschner, T., Dunn, J., Papousek, M., de Boysson-Bardies, B., & Fukui, I. (1989). A cross-language study of prosodic modifications in mothers' and fathers' speech to preverbal infants. *Journal of Child Language, 16*(3), 477–501.

Festinger, L. (1954). A theory of social comparison processes. *Human Relations, 7*(2), 117–140.

George, J. M. (1991). State or trait: Effects of positive mood on prosocial behaviors at work. *Journal of Applied Psychology, 76*(2), 299–307.

Geretsegger, M., Holck, U., & Gold, C. (2012). Randomised controlled trial of improvisational music therapy's effectiveness for children with autism spectrum disorders (TIME-A): Study protocol. *BMC Pediatrics, 12*(1), 2.

Gold, C., Wigram, T., & Elefant, C. (2006). Music therapy for autistic spectrum disorder. *Cochrane Database Systematic Reviews*, 2. https://www.cochrane.org/CD004381/BEHAV_music-therapy-people-autism-spectrum-disorder

Goldin-Meadow, S. (1999). The role of gesture in communication and thinking. *Trends in Cognitive Sciences, 3*(11), 419–429.

Good, A., & Russo, F. A. (2016). Singing promotes cooperation in a diverse group of children. *Social Psychology, 47*, 340–344. https://doi.org/10.1027/1864-9335/a000282

Gooding, L. F. (2011). The effect of a music therapy social skills training program on improving social competence in children and adolescents with social skills deficits. *Journal of Music Therapy, 48*(4), 440–462.

Gregory, A. H., Worrall, L., & Sarge, A. (1996). The development of emotional responses to music in young children. *Motivation and Emotion, 20*(4), 341–348.

Habibi, A., Ilari, B., Crimi, K., Metke, M., Kaplan, J. T., Joshi, A. A., . . . Haldar, & J. P. (2014). An equal start: absence of group differences in cognitive, social, and neural measures prior to music or sports training in children. *Frontiers in Human Neuroscience, 8*, 1–11. https://doi.org/10.3389/fnhum.2014.00690

Habibi, A., Cahn, B. R., Damasio, A., & Damasio, H. (2016). Neural correlates of accelerated auditory processing in children engaged in music training. *Developmental Cognitive Neuroscience, 21*, 1–14.

Hallam, S. (2010). The power of music: Its impact on the intellectual, social and personal development of children and young people. *International Journal of Music Education, 28*(3), 269–289.

Hallam, S., Price, J., & Katsarou, G. (2002). The effects of background music on primary school pupils' task performance. *Educational Studies, 28*(2), 111–122.

Hardy, M. W., & LaGasse, A. B. (2013). Rhythm, movement, and autism: Using rhythmic rehabilitation research as a model for autism. *Frontiers in Integrative Neuroscience, 7*, 1–9. https://doi.org/10.3389/fnint.2013.00019

Hilliard, R. E. (2001). The effects of music therapy-based bereavement groups on mood and behavior of grieving children: A pilot study. *Journal of Music Therapy, 38*(4), 291–306.

Ho, Y.-C., Cheung, M.-C., & Chan, A. S. (2003). Music training improves verbal but not visual memory: Cross-sectional and longitudinal explorations in children. *Neuropsychology, 17*(3), 439.

Holmes, J. (1993). *John Bowlby and attachment theory*. Psychology Press.

Hooper, J., & Lindsay, B. (1990). Music and the mentally handicapped—The effect of music on anxiety. *Journal of British Music Therapy, 4*(2), 19–26.

Huron, D. (2001). Is music an evolutionary adaptation? *Annals of the New York Academy of Sciences, 930*(1), 43–61.

Iacoboni, M., Woods, R. P., Brass, M., Bekkering, H., Mazziotta, J. C., & Rizzolatti, G. (1999). Cortical mechanisms of human imitation. *Science 286*, 2526–2528.

Ilari, B., Fesjian, C., & Habibi, A. (2018). Entrainment, theory of mind, and prosociality in child musicians. *Music & Science, 1*, 1–11.

Isen, A. M., & Labroo, A. A. (2003). Some ways in which positive affect facilitates decision making and judgment. In S. L. Schneider & J. Shanteau (Eds.), *Emerging perspectives on judgment and decision research* (pp. 365–393). Cambridge University Press.

Janzen, T. B., Thompson, W. F., & Ranvaud, R. (2014). A developmental study of the effect of music training on timed movements. *Frontiers in Human Neuroscience, 8*, 1–7. https://doi.org/10.3389/fnhum.2014.00801

Jaschke, A. C., Honing, H., & Scherder, E. J. (2018). Longitudinal analysis of music education on executive functions in primary school children. *Frontiers in Neuroscience, 12*, 1–11. https://doi.org/10.3389/fnins.2018.00103

Juslin, P. N., & Sloboda, J. A. (2001). *Music and emotion: Theory and research*. Oxford University Press.

Juslin, P. N., & Sloboda, J. (2011). *Handbook of music and emotion: Theory, research, applications*. Oxford University Press.

Kersten, L. (2015). Music and cognitive extension. *Empirical Musicology Review, 9*(3-4), 193–202.

Keysers, C., Kohler, E., Umiltà, M. A., Nanetti, L., Fogassi, L., & Gallese, V. (2003). Audiovisual mirror neurons and action recognition. *Experimental Brain Research, 153*(4), 628–636.

Kim, J., Wigram, T., & Gold, C. (2008). The effects of improvisational music therapy on joint attention behaviors in autistic children: A randomized controlled study. *Journal of Autism and Developmental Disorders, 38*(9), 1758–1766.

Kim, J., Wigram, T., & Gold, C. (2009). Emotional, motivational and interpersonal responsiveness of children with autism in improvisational music therapy. *Autism, 13*(4), 389–409.

Kirschner, S., & Tomasello, M. (2009). Joint drumming: Social context facilitates synchronization in preschool children. *Journal of Experimental Child Psychology, 102*(3), 299–314.

Kirschner, S., & Tomasello, M. (2010). Joint music making promotes prosocial behavior in 4-year-old children. *Evolution and Human Behavior, 31*(5), 354–364.

Kohler, E., Keysers, C., Umilta, M. A., Fogassi, L., Gallese, V., & Rizzolatti, G. (2002). Hearing sounds, understanding actions: Action representation in mirror neurons. *Science, 297*(5582), 846–848.

Koyama, T., McHaffie, J. G., Laurienti, P. J., & Coghill, R. C. (2005). The subjective experience of pain: Where expectations become reality. *Proceedings of the National Academy of Sciences of the United States of America, 102*(36), 12950–12955.

Kraus, N., & Chandrasekaran, B. (2010). Music training for the development of auditory skills. *Nature Reviews Neuroscience, 11*(8), 599.

Kwekkeboom, K. L. (2003). Music versus distraction for procedural pain and anxiety in patients with cancer. *The Oncology nursing forum, 30*(3), 433–440. https://doi.org/10.1188/03.ONF.

LaGasse, A. B. (2017). Social outcomes in children with autism spectrum disorder: A review of music therapy outcomes. *Patient Related Outcome Measures, 8*, 23–32.

Lamont, A. (2009). Music in the school years. Hallam, S., Cross, I., & Thaut, M. (Eds.). *The Oxford handbook of music psychology* (pp. 235–243). Oxford University Press.

Lim, H. A., & Draper, E. (2011). The effects of music therapy incorporated with applied behavior analysis verbal behavior approach for children with autism spectrum disorders. *Journal of Music Therapy, 48*(4), 532–550.

Lindblad, F., Hogmark, Å., & Theorell, T. (2007). Music intervention for 5th and 6th graders—Effects on development and cortisol secretion. *Stress and Health, 23*(1), 9–14.

Lively, S. E., Logan, J. S., & Pisoni, D. B. (1993). Training Japanese listeners to identify English/r/and/l/. II: The role of phonetic environment and talker variability in learning new perceptual categories. *The Journal of the Acoustical Society of America, 94*(3), 1242–1255.

Loewenstein, G., & Lerner, J. S. (2003). The role of affect in decision making. In R. H. Goldsmith Davidson & K. Scherer (Eds.), *Handbook of affective science* (pp. 619–642). Oxford University Press.

Marsh, K., & Young, S. (2006). Musical play. In G. McPherson, (Ed.), *The child as musician: A handbook of musical development*, 289–310.

Magne, C., Schön, D., & Besson, M. (2006). Musician children detect pitch violations in both music and language better than nonmusician children: Behavioral and electrophysiological approaches. *Journal of Cognitive Neuroscience, 18*(2), 199–211.

Mehr, S., Schachner, A., Katz, R., & Spelke, E. (2013). Two randomized trials provide no consistent evidence for nonmusical cognitive benefits of brief preschool music enrichment. *PLoS ONE 8*(12), e82007.

Mehr, S. A., Song, L. A., & Spelke, E. S. (2016). For 5-month-old infants, melodies are social. *Psychological Science, 27*(4), 486–501.

Merker, B. (2000). Synchronous chorusing and human origins. In N. L. Wallin, B. Merker, & S. Brown (Eds.), *The origins of music* (pp. 315–327). The MIT Press.

Miladinia, M., Baraz, S., & Zarea, K. (2016). Controlling acute post-operative pain in Iranian children with using of music therapy. *International Journal of Pediatrics, 4*(5), 1725–1730.

Molnar-Szakacs, I., & Overy, K. (2006). Music and mirror neurons: From motion to 'e'motion. *Social Cognitive and Affective Neuroscience, 1*(3), 235–241.

Moore, R. C. (2017). *Childhood's domain: Play and place in child development* (Vol. 6). Routledge.

Moreno, S. (2009). Can music influence language and cognition? *Contemporary Music Review, 28*(3), 329–345.

Moreno, S., Bialystok, E., Barac, R., Schellenberg, E. G., Cepeda, N. J., & Chau, T. (2011). Short-term music training enhances verbal intelligence and executive function. *Psychological Science, 22*(11), 1425–1433.

Mosing, M. A., Madison, G., Pedersen, N. L., & Ullén, F. (2016). Investigating cognitive transfer within the framework of music practice: Genetic pleiotropy rather than causality. *Developmental Science, 19*(3), 504–512.

Nguyen, T. N., Nilsson, S., Hellström, A.-L., & Bengtson, A. (2010). Music therapy to reduce pain and anxiety in children with cancer undergoing lumbar puncture: A randomized clinical trial. *Journal of Pediatric Oncology Nursing, 27*(3), 146–155.

Norton, A., Winner, E., Cronin, K., Overy, K., Lee, D. J., & Schlaug, G. (2005). Are there preexisting neural, cognitive, or motoric markers for musical ability? *Brain and Cognition, 59*(2), 124–134.

Odell, H. (1988). A music therapy approach in mental health. *Psychology of Music, 16*(1), 52–61.

Oldfield, A. (2006). *Interactive music therapy: A positive approach: Music therapy at a child development centre.* Jessica Kingsley Publishers.

Papalia, D. E., Olds, S. W., & Feldman, R. D. (2007). *Human development.* McGraw-Hill.

Papoušek, H. (1996). Musicality in infancy research: Biological and cultural origins of early musicality. In I. Deliège & J. A. Sloboda (Eds.), *Musical beginnings: Origins and development of musical competence* (pp. 37–55), Oxford University Press.

Papoušek, M., & Papoušek, H. (1981). Musical elements in the infant's vocalization: Their significance for communication, cognition, and creativity. *Advances in Infancy Research 1,* 163–224.

Paul, S., & Ramsey, D. (2000). Music therapy in physical medicine and rehabilitation. *Australian Occupational Therapy Journal, 47*(3), 111–118.

Pavlicevic, M. (1999). *Music therapy: Intimate notes.* Jessica Kingsley Publishers.

Pavlicevic, M. (2003). *Groups in music: Strategies from music therapy.* Jessica Kingsley Publishers.

Perry, P. (2020). *The book you wish your parents had read:(and your children will be glad that you did).* Penguin.

Phillips, D. A., & Shonkoff, J. P. (2000). *From neurons to neighborhoods: The science of early childhood development*: National Academies Press.

Phillips-Silver, J., & Keller, P. (2012). Searching for roots of entrainment and joint action in early musical interactions. *Frontiers in Human Neuroscience, 6,* 1–11. https://doi.org/10.3389/fnhum.2012.00026

Piaget, J., & Inhelder, B. (2008). *The psychology of the child.* Basic Books.

Pitts, S. E. (2007). Anything goes: A case study of extra-curricular musical participation in an English secondary school. *Music Education Research, 9*(1), 145–165.

Porter, S., McConnell, T., McLaughlin, K., Lynn, F., Cardwell, C., Braiden, H. J., . . . & Holmes, V. (2017). Music therapy for children and adolescents with behavioural and emotional problems: A randomised controlled trial. *Journal of Child Psychology and Psychiatry, 58*(5), 586–594.

Portowitz, A., Lichtenstein, O., Egorova, L., & Brand, E. (2009). Underlying mechanisms linking music education and cognitive modifiability. *Research Studies in Music Education, 31*(2), 107–128.

Rabinowitch, T.-C., Cross, I., & Burnard, P. (2013). Long-term musical group interaction has a positive influence on empathy in children. *Psychology of Music, 41*(4), 484–498.

Rabinowitch, T. C., & Knafo-Noam, A. (2015). Synchronous rhythmic interaction enhances children's perceived similarity and closeness towards each other. *PLOS one, 10*(4), e0120878.

Rabinowitch, T. C., & Meltzoff, A. N. (2017a). Joint rhythmic movement increases 4-year-old children's prosocial sharing and fairness toward peers. *Frontiers inpsychology, 8,* 1–9. https://doi.org/10.3389/fpsyg.2017.01050.

Rabinowitch, T. C., & Meltzoff, A. N. (2017b). Synchronized movement experience enhances peer cooperation in preschool children. *Journal of Experimental Child Psychology, 160,* 21–32.

Rickson, D. J. (2006). Instructional and improvisational models of music therapy with adolescents who have attention deficit hyperactivity disorder (ADHD): A comparison of the effects on motor impulsivity. *Journal of Music Therapy, 43*(1), 39–62.

Rizzolatti, G., & Craighero, L. (2004). The mirror-neuron system. *Annual Review of Neuroscience, 27,* 169–192.

Robarts, J. (2006). Music therapy with sexually abused children. *Clinical Child Psychology and Psychiatry, 11*(2), 249–269.

Ruud, E. (2008). Music in therapy: Increasing possibilities for action. *Music and Arts in Action 1*(1), 46–60.

Sala, G., & Gobet, F. (2017). When the music's over: Does music skill transfer to children's and young adolescents' cognitive and academic skills? A meta-analysis. *Educational Research Review, 20*, 55–67.

Schellenberg, E. G. (2005). Music and cognitive abilities. *Current Directions in Psychological Science, 14*(6), 317–320.

Schellenberg, E. G. (2006). Long-term positive associations between music lessons and IQ. *Journal of Educational Psychology, 98*(2), 457–468.

Schellenberg, E. G., & Hallam, S. (2005). Music listening and cognitive abilities in 10- and 11-year-olds: The blur effect. *Annals of the New York Academy of Sciences, 1060*(1), 202–209.

Schellenberg, E. G., & Mankarious, M. (2012). Music training and emotion comprehension in childhood. *Emotion, 12*(5), 887–891.

Schellenberg, E. G., & Weiss, M. W. (2013). Music and cognitive abilities. In Diana Deutsch (Ed.), *The psychology of music* (3rd ed.), (pp. 499–550): Elsevier.

Schlaug, G., Norton, A., Overy, K., & Winner, E. (2005). Effects of music training on the child's brain and cognitive development. *Annals of the New York Academy of Sciences, 1060*(1), 219–230. https://doi.org/10.1196/annals.1360.015.

Shaffer, D. R., & Kipp, K. (2013). *Developmental psychology: Childhood and adolescence.* Cengage Learning.

Small, C. (2011). *Musicking: The meanings of performing and listening.* Wesleyan University Press.

Smoski, W. J., Brunt, M. A., & Tannahill, J. C. (1992). Listening characteristics of children with central auditory processing disorders. *Language, Speech, and Hearing Services in Schools, 23*(2), 145–152.

Snyder, B. (2000). *Music and memory: An introduction.* MIT Press.

Spiro, N., & Himberg, T. (2016). Analysing change in music therapy interactions of children with communication difficulties. *Philosophical transactions of the Royal Society of London. Series B, Biological sciences, 371*(1693), 20150374. https://doi.org/10.1098/rstb.2015.0374

Spychiger, M., Patry, J. Lauper, G., Zimmerman, E., & Weber, E. (1993). Does more music teaching lead to a better social climate. In R. Olechowski & G. Svik (Eds.), *Experimental research in teaching and learning.* Bern, Peter Lang.

Swaminathan, S., & Schellenberg, E. G. (2016). Music training. In T. Strobach & J. Karbach (Eds.), *Cognitive training: An overview of features and applications* (pp. 137–144). Springer International Publishing AG.

Swaminathan, S., Schellenberg, E. G., & Khalil, S. (2017). Revisiting the association between music lessons and intelligence: Training effects or music aptitude? *Intelligence, 62*, 119–124.

Sward, R. (1989). Band is a family. *Today's Music Educator*, Winter, 26–27 .

Theorell, T., Lennartsson, A. K., Madison, G., Mosing, M., & Ullén, F. (2015). Predictors of continued playing or singing—From childhood and adolescence to adult years. *Acta Paediatrica, 104*(3), 274–284.

Tomaino, C. M. (2012). Effective music therapy techniques in the treatment of nonfluent aphasia. *Annals of the New York Academy of Sciences, 1252*(1), 312–317.

Trevarthen, C., & Aitken, K. J. (2001). Infant intersubjectivity: Research, theory, and clinical applications. *The Journal of Child Psychology and Psychiatry and Allied Disciplines, 42*(1), 3–48.

Tudge, J., & Rogoff, B. (1999). Peer influences on cognitive development: Piagetian and Vygotskian perspectives. In P. Lloyd & C. Fernyhough (Eds.), *Lev Vygotsky: Critical assessments. Vol. 3. The zone of proximal development* (pp. 32–56). Routledge.

Tunçgenç, B., & Cohen, E. (2016). Movement synchrony forges social bonds across group divides. *Frontiers in Psychology, 7*, 1–12. https://doi.org/10.3389/fpsyg.2016.00782

Tunçgenç, B., & Cohen, E. (2018). Interpersonal movement synchrony facilitates pro-social behavior in children's peer-play. *Developmental Science, 21*(1), 1–9.

Turino, T. (2008). *Music as social life: The politics of participation*: University of Chicago Press.

Uggla, L., Bonde, L., Svahn, B., Remberger, M., Wrangsjö, B., & Gustafsson, B. (2016). Music therapy can lower the heart rates of severely sick children. *Acta Pædiatrica, 105*(10), 1225–1230.

Vaiouli, P., Grimmet, K., & Ruich, L. J. (2015). 'Bill is now singing': Joint engagement and the emergence of social communication of three young children with autism. *Autism, 19*(1), 73–83.

Watkins, K. E., Strafella, A. P., & Paus, T. (2003). Seeing and hearing speech excites the motor system involved in speech production. *Neuropsychologia, 41*(8), 989–994.

Welch, G., Ockelford, A., Carter, F.-C., Zimmermann, S.-A., & Himonides, E. (2009). Sounds of intent: Mapping musical behaviour and development in children and young people with complex needs. *Psychology of Music, 37*(3), 348–370.

Wheeler, B. L. (2005). Music therapy research. In J. Edwards (Ed.), *The Oxford handbook of music therapy* (pp. 709–719). Oxford University Press.

Wigram, T. (2004). *Improvisation: Methods and techniques for music therapy clinicians, educators, and students*: Jessica Kingsley Publishers.

Wu, L., Yu, H., & Liu, Y. (2008). Combined treatment using acupuncture and music therapy on children with cerebral palsy. *Neural Regeneration Research, 3*(6), 694–696.

Young, K. D. (2005). Pediatric procedural pain. *Annals of Emergency Medicine, 45*(2), 160–171.

Zatorre, R. J., Chen, J. L., & Penhune, V. B. (2007). When the brain plays music: auditory— Motor interactions in music perception and production. *Nature Reviews Neuroscience, 8*(7), 547.

3
Musical care in adolescence
Supporting healthy musical identities and uses of music

Suvi Saarikallio and Katrina Skewes McFerran

Introduction

Adolescence is the critical step towards independence and adult identity (World Health Organization, 2020a). Adolescence—referring to ages 10 to 19 years—is the time of great passion, potential, and growth, yet also of great vulnerability. The young generation holds the power to renew societies, but the developmental path of adolescents to empowerment, maturity, and wisdom is not always so smooth. Each young person has to find their steps to adult identity and negotiate their sense of belonging, relationships, values, and independence. At the same time, the modern world is filled with stressors such as inequality, immigration, and climate change, which accelerate paths towards anxiety, depression, aggression, and marginalization. In Europe, 25% of young people (and 44% of migrant young people born outside of the European Union) are at risk of poverty or social exclusion (Eurostat, 2019), which feeds adverse mental health outcomes, non-communicable diseases and, in extreme cases, suicide (AYPH: Association for Young People's Health, 2017). As an age group, adolescents are particularly vulnerable to developing mental disorders (World Health Organization, 2020b). Not always are the resources of adolescents in line with the demands they face, and this misalignment can cause severe stress and insecurity.

What kind of resources, then, in this modern world would best support youth empowerment and healthy development? How could we help adolescents to find their place and to flourish? The 2010s into the 2020s have witnessed a boom of interest in understanding the potential of music to support health and well-being (MacDonald et al., 2011) and have seen efforts to develop an evidence base for the positive health impacts of music and art (for example, Fancourt & Finn, 2019). Many of the underlying mechanisms of why music functions positively in people's lives are shared across all age groups. While acknowledging this point, we also wish in this chapter to highlight the special nature of adolescence, aiming to provide insight into how and why music is perhaps a well-suited companion particularly to this sensitive phase of life.

It has been proposed that a passion for popular music is the clearest marker of adolescence (Christenson & Roberts, 1998). Researchers have stressed that music is not just entertainment for adolescents but also actually holds the potential to support

Suvi Saarikallio and Katrina Skewes McFerran, *Musical care in adolescence* In: *Collaborative Insights*. Edited by: Neta Spiro and Katie Rose M. Sanfilippo, Oxford University Press. © Oxford University Press 2022. DOI: 10.1093/oso/9780197535011.003.0004 their most fundamental developmental and psychological needs, including identity development and emotional self-regulation (Laiho, 2004; Miranda, 2013; North et al., 2000; Saarikallio, 2019c, as also discussed in the Musical care in childhood chapter). The relatedness of music to both identity (MacDonald et al., 2017) and emotions (Juslin & Sloboda, 2010) has received wide research attention in recent years. These aspects are also fundamental to adolescents, in terms of their development in general, and in terms of supporting their health and well-being in particular. For instance, research on youth development shows that one of the critical protective factors buffering against social and mental problems on a journey towards adulthood is the adaptive development of their social-emotional skills (Eisenberg & Fabes, 1999; Zeman et al., 2006). In this chapter we discuss the role of music as a resource that can support these critical elements of positive adolescent development.

Finally, this chapter embraces interdisciplinary dialogue on this topic. Research in music psychology has typically focused on the influence of music on emotions and an interest in *why* music helps. Music therapists, however, have tended to prioritize the emotional experience of young people in their musical encounter, focusing on *how* music helps. Music sociologists have been more focused on the ways in which adolescents engage with music in different contexts, placing a firmer emphasis on *where* music helps. And sometimes these perspectives have been brought together. For example, McFerran (2020) has considered this important contextualization in describing how adolescents experience music therapy in different contexts, bringing together some of these influences. In this chapter, we follow the example of our edited *Handbook of Music, Adolescents, and Wellbeing* (McFerran et al., 2019) and bridge perspectives from music psychology, music therapy, music education, and music sociology in order to provide an interdisciplinary view of why, how, and where musical care plays a role in adolescent development. In this chapter, musical care is understood to refer to the ways in which adolescents, given the importance of agency during this life stage, appropriate the affordances of music (Ansdell & DeNora, 2015) for their own well-being.

We, the authors, began to work together to understand how music therapy theory could ground and strengthen music psychology research, and how music psychology research could provide foundations for deepening understandings of music therapy. Katrina McFerran is a music therapy professor whose expertise is grounded in her practice with young people in mental and physical health contexts, as well as in schools. Suvi Saarikallio's research in music psychology focuses on the primary psychological functions of music for adolescents: identity, agency, and interpersonal relationships and how these intersect with emotions.

In this chapter, we will explore the following themes as one way of examining how music can be used to support healthy musical identities and uses of music. First, the powerful impact of music on our emotions and *musical care for emotional development and self-regulation* in adolescence will be presented. Next, we will examine *musical care in personal and social identity*, wherein we will explore music as an expression of, and development of, identity and a way to connect. Thereafter, we bring out the notion that while being a powerful resource, music is not always used in helpful ways and young people may also need support and guidance in their music use. Thus, the *unhelpful uses of music in adolescence* will be explored as well as *promoting intentional uses of musical care of adolescents in practice*. Finally, future directions of interdisciplinary research in this area are explored.

Musical care for emotional development and self-regulation

Theories about the capacity to adaptively manage and utilize emotions typically hold the idea that basic-level skills of emotion recognition and awareness build resources for higher-order skills of self-regulation and social interaction (Denham et al., 2012; Mayer & Salovey, 1997; Van Beveren et al., 2019). In adolescence, many of these critical skills are still developing. In terms of emotional awareness, the use of emotion words and bodily sensation patterns of emotions gradually develops towards adult-like patterns across ages 6 to 17 years (Hietanen et al., 2016). Some studies suggest that there are even declines during adolescence in the ability for facial emotion recognition (Lawrence et al., 2015; Thomas et al., 2007) and use of emotion words (Baron-Cohen et al., 2010). However, the evidence of this decline is inconclusive (Vetter et al., 2018) and some theorists point to evidence that there is an enormous diversity of emotional development across adults, and that many young people demonstrate more mature emotional capacities than many adults (Epstein, 2007). Nevertheless, research has shown that emotional development is an important area of research and care during adolescence.

The capacity of music to reach emotions has been identified as a central reason for why music is psychologically relevant for people at all ages, as shown throughout the other chapters of this book (Juslin & Laukka, 2004; Juslin & Sloboda, 2010). Yet this capacity is perhaps the case particularly for adolescents, to whom music provides emotional support for a range of core developmental tasks involving identity, close relationships, and growth to independence (Laiho, 2004; Gold et al., 2011). For instance, on the basis of a large survey (N≈2500) among British adolescents North et al. (2000) reported that adolescents valued music for two main reasons: for supporting their identity expression and for satisfying their emotional needs. Through group interviews with 14- to 17-year-olds, Saarikallio and Erkkilä (2007) identified that adolescents actively use music as a tool for their emotional self-regulation, employing a range of regulation strategies from distraction, revival, and strong sensations to processing their personal experiences through mental work and finding solace, comfort, and emotional validation.

Emotional self-regulation (Beauchaine, 2015; Zeman et al., 2006) actively develops during adolescence. Moreover, adolescence may hold challenging moments for self-regulation. For instance, a reduced use of adaptive emotion regulation strategies and an increased use of maladaptive strategies have been reported in adolescents between

12 and 15 years of age (Cracco et al., 2017). Emotional development is also visible at the neural level, with great plasticity and development taking place in brain areas involved in emotional processing (Burnett et al., 2009; Fuhrmann et al., 2015). Overall, emotional development is taking critical steps during the adolescent years. Tools like music that can facilitate the integration of embodied and cognitive levels of the affective knowledge can be very attractive and powerful at this phase of life.

Music has been considered to be communicative and embodied, allowing for the awareness and expression of emotion. Nonverbal communication in music functions across the sensory modalities of sound, touch, and vision utilizing the affective shades and nuances that are shared amongst them. For example, child psychologists Daniel Stern (1999) and Colwyn Trevarthen (Traverthen & Aitken, 2001) have argued that music and art operate through the affective-embodied levels of human experience. Musical sounds function as a bridge between our bodily experiences and the awareness of these experiences (Lesaffre et al., 2017). Similar to communication in music, cognition has also been argued to be embodied. For example, cognition is seen not just to happen in our heads but also to involve the dynamic interaction between bodily and environmental factors (Ward & Stapleton, 2012). This discovery has been summarized in the relatively recent enactive cognition perspective, the 4Es framework: embodied, embedded, enactive, and extended (Newen et al., 2018; Ward & Stapleton, 2012). In music psychotherapy, a type of music therapy, music is considered to provide access to the nonverbal experiences, make the internal external, concretize what we feel inside, and allow fragile experiences to become tangible, understandable, and manageable (Erkkilä et al., 2012; Geipel, 2019). In essence, we can 'offload' part of our affective-cognitive processes onto external resources—including art and music (Krueger, 2014).

Music can provide the 'words' to adolescents' experiences of their daily life. The recent access-awareness-agency (AAA) model of music-based social-emotional competence integrates these arguments to define music as a skill of reaching embodied *access* to, reflective *awareness* of, and sense of *agency* over one's social-emotional experiences (Saarikallio, 2019a). McFerran (2016) compares the ways that music psychologists and music therapists describe working with emotions in ways that encompass the AAA spectrum. She suggests that the music psychology discourse tends to focus on explaining how to manage emotions and their influence, while therapy discourse focuses on recognition and expression of emotions together with the therapist, in musical experiences. Music psychology research has been closely aligned with the general emotional competence literature, which typically focuses on cognitive (e.g., emotion recognition, emotional clarity) and behavioural (self-regulation, use of emotional knowledge) levels of emotional knowing, while the strength of music as an emotional competence, and as a form of therapy, is fundamentally rooted in the capacity of music to ground these 'higher' levels of experience in the embodied level of knowing (McFerran, 2016, Saarikallio, 2019c).

Baltazar and Saarikallio present a model of music listening that includes the interplay of cognitions, feelings, and bodily states (Baltazar, 2019; Baltazar & Saarikallio,

2019). This model of musical affect self-regulation divides between individual-dependent mechanisms (e.g., memories, identification) serving the immersion into cognitive-affective-attentional processing, and feature-dependent mechanisms (e.g., rhythm, contagion) serving repair-distraction-pleasure-oriented regulation (Baltazar & Saarikallio, 2019). Music is indeed a powerful tool both for allowing deep immersion into our inner experiences and for distracting us. Genevieve Dingle (2019) discusses emotional immersion in further detail, arguing that immersion in sadness and anger in the context of music is not necessarily maladaptive and ruminative, but can actually be a process towards feeling better afterwards. Saarikallio (2018) argues that attraction to sad music is partly explained by music being a catalyst for emotional processing: by bridging bodily, symbolic, and cognitive levels of experience. Music speeds up the process of emotion being activated, accepted, and managed, and new meaning-making accessed. Examples of how the capacity of music to reach emotional processing include work with adolescents for violence prevention (Wölfl, 2019) and treatment of depression (Geipel, 2019). Both Geipel and Wölfl elaborate how music can be utilized as an opportunity to express, experience, and regulate emotions non-verbally, as an emotional space of understanding one's feelings, as a bridge of these experiences to verbal communication, and as a tool for gaining insight of one's own and also of others' emotions, behaviours, and needs.

Musical care in personal and social identity

In addition to satisfying emotional needs, North et al. (2000) identified music to be important for adolescents in terms of supporting their identity expression. In the 1980s already, Frith (1981) described how music can serve as a badge of identity for young people and thus launched discussion of the relevance of music as part of youth identity development. Musical identities are currently understood as constantly evolving conceptions about how we perceive ourselves and relate ourselves with the world through music—our musical preferences, meanings, and daily engagements with music (MacDonald et al., 2017). Music is considered as a powerful resource for developing personal and social identity. For instance, the *Handbook of Musical Identities* (MacDonald et al., 2017) offers a wide variety of perspectives to how music functions as a part of identity construction. Meanwhile, authors in the *Handbook of Music, Adolescents, and Wellbeing* discuss this affordance of music particularly for the age group of adolescents. Dave Miranda (2019), a music psychologist, argues that music serves as a reflection of youth personality and Alexandra Lamont and David Hargreaves (2019), researchers in music psychology and music education, emphasize that music functions as a resource for adolescents' social identity construction. The music therapist Elly Scrine (2019) describes music as a tool that helps young people to explore their sexuality, and Viggo Krüger (2019), a musician and music therapist, argues that in child welfare contexts, music can help adolescents to reconstruct a positive identity and restore one's capacity for social participation. In many ways, music is a means both to connect with other adolescents and to help adolescents find the connection to who they are and who they want to become (music therapist P. Derrington, 2019). And when we finally become adults, music is the very tool that provides us a bridge back to our youth identity (music sociologist T. DeNora, 2019).

Why is music such a powerful resource for how adolescents define themselves and how they wish to present themselves to others? Saarikallio (2019b) argues that music is an attractive and important tool for adolescents' identity development because it supports their sense of agency and self-determination. In adolescence, there is a great demand for establishing an adult identity while the range of alternative options for careers, relationships, and world views is broadening (Côté & Levine, 2002): identity construction has become a process of finding one's own path to adulthood, a task that places great demands on the capacity for exercising personal agency (Schwartz et al., 2013). Agency is established as a dialogue of personal capacities and the social, cultural, and environmental structures that both provide support and place limits on agency (Cote & Levine, 2002). In adolescence, many of the major areas of life are still defined and determined by adult guidance, while music and other hobbies provide more freedom for adolescents themselves in determining their goals, modes of action, and criteria for success (Saarikallio, 2019b).

Music can metaphorically be considered as the playground of adolescents. It is not owned by the adults, or the teachers, or the parents, although the adolescent music industry is carefully manicured with multiple invisible adult influences (Nuttal, 2009). Nonetheless, young people experience music as a realm of their own, beyond adult surveillance. This sense of ownership makes music a powerful, and necessary, tool for the developing sense of independence and identity. Modern pedagogy of music education also emphasizes the relevance of involving adolescents themselves as agentic actors of their own learning (Westerlund et al., 2017) and that music education experiences should be supportive of adolescents' basic psychological needs of competence, relatedness, and autonomy (Evans & McPherson, 2017). The combination of music and the range of digital technology and social media are great tools for addressing the voice and the perspectives of adolescents themselves, appreciating and adopting the ways they connect to one another and wish to be heard by others (Cheong-Clinch, 2019; Pluretti & Bobkowski, 2019; Viega, 2019).

Unhelpful uses of music in adolescence

Our recent collaborative research has elaborated on the complex interplay of factors that impact the healthiness of adolescents' music use. Indeed, oftentimes, personal music use supports adolescents' needs for belonging, self-determination, emotional support, and identity formation (Gold et al., 2011; North et al., 2000). However, not all young people are always able to appropriate the positive affordances of music, and those who are struggling may use it for reinforcing more complex moods and emotions, and even end up worsening pathological states. A range of individual factors and specific patterns of (consciously or unconsciously) using music are essentially involved in explaining how music functions as a promoter of or hindrance to health and care. The health-fostering patterns of using music in adolescence involve the experiences discussed previously: the emotion modulation, reflective awareness, and agency. Such patterns of music use can be conceptualized as competencies in the use of music for healthy development.

The ways that adolescents use these competencies are highly varied, however, this variance canvasses the ways that music is appropriated towards emotional development, self-regulation, and personal and social identity formation. In a large qualitative investigation of the ways young people use music, we identified four categories described by the participants—including managing relationships, promoting coping, impacting mood, and expressing identity (McFerran & Saarikallio, 2013). Within each of those major categories there were a number of subcategories, some that described healthy uses of music, and others that described less helpful strategies. Until that time, the examination of adolescents and music had been either entirely positive with a focus on agency and self-expression, or, judgmental and negative, with a focus on the ways that music could make young people behave badly—labelled problem music (North & Hargreaves, 2008). Our research suggested that young people sometimes used music in ways that were helpful and at other times, the same music could be used in unhelpful ways. This was an intriguing notion that leaped out from our data and led us to reconsider these as distinct ways people use music, and to explore the notion more carefully.

Drawing on the words of the 50 young Australians who participated in the qualitative study that underpinned our theory construction, we then developed a list of questions designed for young people to complete. These questions canvassed both healthy and unhealthy uses of music, with the dimensions of unhealthy use including rumination and avoidance. After a number of experiments, the final scale (Healthy Unhealthy Music Scale, or HUMS) included 13 items, consisting of five healthy and eight unhealthy items, as seen in the following list (Saarikallio et al., 2015).

HUMS Unhealthy

- When I listen to music, I get stuck in bad memories.
- I like to listen to songs over and over even though it makes me feel worse.
- It can be hard to stop listening to music.
- I hide in my music because nobody understands me, and it blocks people out.
- When I try to use music to feel better, I actually end up feeling worse.
- Music gives me an excuse not to face up to the real world.
- Music makes me feel bad about who I am.
- Music leads me to do things I shouldn't do.

HUMS Healthy:

- I feel happier after playing or listening to music.
- Music gives me the energy to get going.

- When I'm feeling tense or tired in my body, music helps me to relax.
- Music helps me to relax.
- Music helps me to connect with other people who are like me.

Adolescents (aged 13–20) were asked to rate themselves on a Likert scale of 1–5 (never–rarely–sometimes–often–always). Although these questions captured the main ways that adolescents talked about using music, their responses did not mean that they were able to recognize unhealthy uses immediately. We had realized in the initial interviews from the qualitative study that only after probing would adolescents describe unhelpful outcomes from engaging with music. Their initial self-report tended to be exceedingly positive, and only when encouraged would they begin to reflect, 'Well, there was this one time where I felt much worse afterwards.' Thus, we recognized that using music to intensify negative emotional states through rumination and isolation was one part of unconscious patterns of behaviour. And thus, our focus moved to increasing intentional uses of music with adolescents.

Promoting intentional uses of musical care in adolescence in practice

Although adolescents do tend to use music to make themselves feel better when they are well (Saarikallio & Erkkilä, 2007), our collaborative work has suggested that patterns of music use can change during periods of unhappiness and depression. For example, we have observed that during these times, adolescents seemed to believe that their music was going to continue to make them feel better, as it had done during easier times. Therefore, they continued to rely on music, as though it had carried the agency for their state, rather than identifying themselves as the protagonist (Cheong-Clinch & McFerran, 2016). Within music therapy, we have identified a number of ways to support adolescents in owning their own power under these new conditions, and working with adolescents in reconstructing their musical identity was particularly helpful for adolescents with psychosis and schizophrenia diagnoses (Hense & McFerran, 2017). However, we also learned that people who were in an acute stage of their mental illness were not able to use cognitive reframing and recognition of patterns of behaviour (Hense et al., 2018) to think about their uses of music. In these cases, music-making and other music therapy methods that focused on the here and now were more engaging and appreciated by adolescents.

With this increased clarity about the importance of cognitive functioning for recognizing unhealthy patterns of music use and increasing healthy uses, we began to develop a brief intervention designed for adolescents struggling with anxiety and depression. In this intervention (McFerran et al., 2018), the questions developed for the HUMS were used as conversational prompts, designed to support shared music listening and playlist construction. The music therapist would engage in conversations about preferred music and ask about how the adolescent felt before and after—increasing awareness of the ways that music selections could prompt emotional movement in various directions. Together, the therapist and adolescent would identify songs that led to positive feelings and those that prompted negative feelings. The ISO Principle—a music therapy technique wherein music is first matched with a client's mood and gradually altered to reach a new, desired mood state (Davis et al., 2008)—was then used to help construct playlists that began with the more difficult emotional states and used a sequence of songs selected by the adolescent to move towards preferred states of being. All songs were selected from within the adolescent's preferred repertoire, usually carried on their mobile devices, and conversations supported increased understanding by the adolescent.

The Intentional Uses of Music (Hense et al., 2018) study showed us that adolescents who were depressed seemed to have minimal insight into their patterns of music use, but that they were very interested to explore new ways of using music. After being involved in only one or two sessions, the majority of adolescents described how, as a result of the intervention, they could actively use music to promote their own personal development rather than positioning themselves as passive recipients of the effect of music. More than half of the adolescents described changes in their ways of using music, either being more careful about their selections at certain times, or actively using playlists at difficult times. Some labelled their playlists as 'Reflective' or 'Boss', and others used them for mood or energy management.

In this mixed methods study, we also collected quantitative data on the levels of distress experienced by participants. The improvements in levels of distress were noteworthy. Although the number of participants who completed both pre- and post-tests meant that probability calculations were too unreliable, in real terms, all participants rated themselves as experiencing a decrease from pre- to post-intervention. This combination of increased sense of agency, changed uses of music, and improvements on distress ratings provided positive evidence that raising awareness in adolescents about their uses of music could be helpful.

On the basis of our experience, our best scientific research has often been motivated by practical, clinical insight and, in turn, our most successful clinical work has often been guided by our research findings. The relationship between music psychology and music therapy is often more of an overlap than a clear distinction. Yet, music psychologists are generally not focused on the application of ideas in practice, but rather on understanding how music can affect well-being. Music therapists can use those insights but need to adapt them significantly to meet the needs of individuals rather than the conglomerate image people might have of the 'adolescent'. This tailoring of music interventions is one example of how musical care is practiced with adolescents who have mental and physical health challenges, and who are struggling during this important transitional stage of life.

Future directions

There are many directions that interdisciplinary practice and research in musical care in adolescence could take. These will always be shaped by the particular histories and contexts of the researchers themselves. The following offers some of our ideas in this area, with an emphasis on practice with young individuals and groups, broadly ranging from clinical care to social work and educational contexts.

First, at a practical level, the realization that adolescents often adopt a passive stance to their music listening, and position themselves as a passive recipient has important implications for practice. Music therapists should always ask about adolescents' own uses of music, with a particular awareness of ruminative and isolating patterns of music use if they are struggling with depression. This approach should be paired with a recognition that this way of intensifying states through music is often unconscious and needs to be gently pursued, since many adolescents have already experienced being told to 'stop' listening. Indeed, schools and mental health institutions may have censorship policies or practices that limit adolescents' freedom for music listening (Kallio, 2017).

Second, using music listening as an important method for working with adolescents is clarified through this exploration of how important music is to adolescents. This clarification is of great relevance to all practical work, from therapy to education. Although it is possible to avoid the associations of preferred music by focusing on music creation—either through composition or improvisation—doing so ignores adolescents' passion for their music. We have outlined how music is continually found to be of enormous significance to adolescents, and how it can be used as a resource (Rolvjsord, 2006, 2010), rather than ignored. To include music that adolescents themselves listen to in our practices with them is to include their personal, social, sexual, and cultural identities, values, and meanings. To do so requires sensitivity yet offers great potential.

Third, music can be used preventatively in non-medical contexts. For example, increasing awareness of the ways that music choices can be more intentional is an excellent basis for classroom-based well-being activities. We have observed how the HUMS can be integrated into classrooms by teachers and other well-being professionals, through discussions that concern the items in relation to the adolescents' own music uses. HUMS items offer an engaging way of raising awareness about the power of music and how to use it for helpful, not unhealthy, outcomes.

Making young people aware of the power of music helps them become more conscious of how important their music selections are, in different moods and on different days, and how those selections can have a wide-scale impact. Many web-based applications have been designed for this purpose, but most lack the nuance of being able to draw out conscious awareness. Instead, they tend to reinforce the idea that music is the bearer of agency. Our findings on this concept have been clear. Music is a way to empower youth to have more agency, to know that their music selections do make a difference, and to realize that they can enjoy music across a range of moods and states in ways that will promote their well-being. Yet, adolescents sometimes need support in realizing how they use music and how they could use music even better.

Music therapists and other health, education, and community welfare professionals working with music and adolescents can function as guides who raise awareness and encourage increased consciousness about how music works. Adolescents can be supported to take agency and ownership of the impacts of their personal music engagement. Doing so can lead to the re-establishment of healthy musical identities and habits. Considering the eminent role of music in the lives of adolescents, opportunities to dialogue with the very use of music by adolescents themselves can be seen as a highly meaningful, efficient, and empowering form of musical care, applicable for a range of contexts from educational and preventive settings to the clinical ones.

Conclusion

The capacity to support the healthy growth of the young generation is of essence to all societies. In Europe, for instance, the European Union youth strategy drafted for 2019–2027 focuses on three keywords—engage, connect, and empower—in order to ensure that all young people would have the necessary resources to take part in the society (European Commission, 2018). We believe that music and musical care have a lot to offer to this shared endeavour, perhaps more than is currently been understood. The relationship between adolescents and music will continue to hold the attention of researchers for many decades to come. With the influx of new technologies making music more accessible, there has been an ever-increasing diversity in adolescents' uses of music. This increase means that we can also expand our repertoire of musical care. Importantly, these affordances can be both positive and negative, helpful and unhelpful, healthy and unhealthy. Drawing mutually from research and clinical practice, we will continue to create new knowledge and insight on how musical care can best support youth empowerment and health.

References

Ansdell, G., & DeNora, T. (2015). *Musical pathways in recovery: Community music therapy and mental wellbeing*. Routledge.
AYPH: Association for Young People's Health. (2017). *Why invest in young people's health?*
Baltazar, M. (2019). Musical affect regulation in adolescents: A conceptual model. In K. McFerran, P. Derrington, & S. Saarikallio (Eds.), *Handbook of music, adolescents, and wellbeing* (pp. 65–74). Oxford University Press.
Baltazar, M., & Saarikallio, S. (2019). Strategies and mechanisms in musical affect self-regulation: A new model. *Musicae Scientiae, 23*(2), 177–195. First published online, June 2017.

Baron-Cohen, S., Golan, O., Wheelwright, S., Granader, Y., & Hill, J. (2010). Emotion word comprehension from 4 to 16 years old: A developmental survey. *Frontiers in Evolutionary Neuroscience, 2,* 109.

Beauchaine, T. P. (2015). Future directions in emotion dysregulation and youth psychopathology. *Journal of Clinical Child & Adolescent Psychology, 44*(5), 875–896.

Burnett, S., Bird, G., Moll, J., Frith, C., & Blakemore, S. J. (2009). Development during adolescence of the neural processing of social emotion. *Journal of Cognitive Neuroscience, 21,* 1736–1750.

Cheong-Clinch, C. (2019). My iPod, YouTube and our playlists: Connections made in and beyond therapy. In K. McFerran, P. Derrington, & S. Saarikallio (Eds.), *Handbook of music, adolescents, and wellbeing* (pp. 225–236). Oxford University Press.

Cheong-Clinch, C., & McFerran, K. S. (2016). Musical diaries: Examining the daily preferred music listening of Australian young people with mental illness. *Journal of Applied Youth Studies, 1*(2), 77–94.

Christenson, P. G., & Roberts, D. F. (1998). *It's not only rock & roll: Popular music in the lives of adolescents.* Hampton Press.

Cote, J. E., & Levine, C. G. (2002). *Identity formation, agency, and culture: A social psychological synthesis.* Erlbaum

Cracco, E., Goossens, L., & Braet, C. (2017). Emotion regulation across childhood and adolescence: Evidence for a maladaptive shift in adolescence. *European Child and Adolescent Psychiatry, 26*(8), 909–921.

Davis, W. B., Gfeller, K. E., & Thaut, M. H. (Eds.). (2008). *An introduction to music therapy theory and practice.* American Music Therapy Association.

Denham, S. A., Bassett, H., Mincic, M., Kalb, S., Way, E., Wyatt, T., & Segal, Y. (2012). Social-emotional learning profiles of preschoolers' early school success: A person-centered approach. *Learning and Individual Differences, 22*(2), 178–189.

DeNora, T. (2019). 'For ever piping songs for ever new': The musical teenager and musical inner teenager across the life course. In K. McFerran, P. Derrington, & S. Saarikallio (Eds.), *Handbook of music, adolescents, and wellbeing.* Oxford University Press.

Derrington, P. (2019). 'What's the WiFi code in here?' Connecting with adolescents in music therapy. In K. McFerran, P. Derrington, & S. Saarikallio (Eds.), *Handbook of music, adolescents, and wellbeing* (pp. 165–174). Oxford University Press.

Dingle, G. (2019). Young people's uses of music for emotional immersion. In K. McFerran, P. Derrington, & S. Saarikallio (Eds.), *Handbook of music, adolescents, and wellbeing* (pp. 25–38). Oxford University Press.

Eisenberg, N., & Fabes, R. A. (1999). Emotion, emotion-related regulation, and quality of socioemotional functioning. In L. Balter & C. Tamis-LeMonda (Eds.), *Child psychology: A handbook of contemporary issues* (pp. 318–335). Psychology Press.

Erkkilä, J., Ala-Ruona, E., Punkanen, M., & Fachner, J. (2012). Creativity in improvisational, psychodynamic music therapy. In D. Hargreaves, D. Miell, & R. MacDonald (Eds.), *Musical imaginations: Multidisciplinary perspectives on creativity, performance and perception* (pp. 414–428). Oxford University Press.

Epstein, R. (2007). *The case against adolescence: Rediscovering the adult in every teen.* Quill Driver Books/Word Dancer Press.

European Commission, Directorate-General for Education, Youth, Sport and Culture. (2018). *Communication from the commission to the European Parliament, the European Council, the European Economic and Social Committee and the Committee of the Regions—Engaging, connecting and empowering young people: A new EU youth strategy.* https://eur-lex.europa.eu/legal-content/en/ALL/?uri=CELEX:52018DC0269

Eurostat. (2019). *Statistics on young people neither in employment nor in education or training.* https://Ec.europa.eu/eurostat/statistics-explained/index.php?title=Statistics_on_young_ people_neither_in_employment_nor_in_education_or_training#Young_people_neither_in_employment_nor_in_education_or_training

Evans, P., & McPherson, G. (2017). Processes of musical identity consolidation during adolescence. In R. MacDonald, D. J. Hargreaves, & D. Miell (Eds.), *Handbook of musical identities* (pp. 213–231). Oxford University Press.

Fancourt, D., & Finn, S. (2019). *What is the evidence on the role of the arts in improving health and well-being? A scoping review* (Health Evidence Network synthesis report 67). WHO Regional Office for Europe.

Frith, S. (1981). *Sound effects: Youth, leisure and the politics of rock 'n' roll.* Pantheon.

Fuhrmann, D., Knoll, L. J., & Blakemore, S. J. (2015). Adolescence as a sensitive period of brain development. *Trends in Cognitive Sciences, 19*(10), 558–566.

Geipel., J. (2019). Between down in the dumps and over the moon: Music therapy for young people with depression. In K. McFerran, P. Derrington, & S. Saarikallio (Eds.), *Handbook of music, adolescents, and wellbeing* (pp. 53–64). Oxford University Press.

Gold, C., Saarikallio, S. H., & McFerran, K. (2011). Music therapy. In R. J. Levesque (Ed.), *Encyclopedia of adolescence* (pp. 1826–1834). Springer.

Hietanen, J. K., Glerean, E., Hari., R., & Nummenmaa, L. (2016). Bodily maps of emotions across child development. *Developmental Science, 19*(6):1111–1118, Epub 2016 Feb 21. PMID: 26898716. https://doi.org/10.1111/desc.1238.

Hense, C., & McFerran, K. S. (2017). Promoting young people's musical identities to facilitate recovery from mental illness. *Journal of Youth Studies, 20*(8), 997–1012. https://doi.org/10.1080/13676261.2017.1287888

Hense, C., McFerran, K. S., & Silverman, M. J. (2018). Using the healthy-unhealthy uses of music scale as a single session music therapy intervention on an acute youth mental health inpatient unit. *Music Therapy Perspectives, 36*(2), 267–276. https://doi.org/10.1093/mtp/miy013

Juslin, P. N., & Laukka, P. (2004). Expression, perception, and induction of musical emotions: A review and a questionnaire study of everyday listening. *Journal of New Music Research, 33*(3), 217–238.

Juslin, P. N., & Sloboda, J. A. (Eds.). (2010). *Handbook of music and emotion: Theory, research, applications.* Oxford University Press.

Kallio, A. A. (2017). Popular outsiders: The censorship of popular music in school music education. *Popular Music and Society, 40*(3), 330–344. https://doi.org/10.1080/03007766.2017.1295213

Krueger, J. (2014). Musical manipulations and the emotionally extended mind. *Empirical Musicology Review, 9*(3), 1–5.

Kruger, V. (2019). Music as a structuring resource in identity formation processes by adolescents engaging in music therapy—A case story from a Norwegian child welfare setting: 'Hey ho, let's go' (The Ramones). In K. McFerran, P. Derrington, & S. Saarikallio (Eds.), *Handbook of music, adolescents, and wellbeing* (pp. 127–138). Oxford University Press.

Laiho, S. (2004). The psychological functions of music in adolescence. *Nordic Journal of Music Therapy, 13*(1), 47–63. https://doi.org/10.1080/08098130409478097

Lamont, A., & Hargreaves, D. (2019). Musical preference and social identity in adolescence. In K. McFerran, P. Derrington, & S. Saarikallio (Eds.), *Handbook of music, adolescents, and wellbeing* (pp. 109–118). Oxford University Press.

Lawrence, K., Campbell, R., & Skuse, D. (2015). Age, gender, and puberty influence the development of facial emotion recognition. *Frontiers in Psychology, 6*, 761.

Lesaffre, M., Maes, P., & Leman, M. (Eds.). (2017). *The Routledge companion to embodied music interaction.* Taylor & Francis.

MacDonald, R., Kreuzt, G., & Mitchell, L. (Eds.). (2011). *Music, health and wellbeing.* Oxford University Press.

MacDonald, R., Hargreaves, D. J., & Miell, D. (Eds.). (2017). *Handbook of musical identities.* Oxford University Press.

Mayer, J. D., & Salovey, P. (1997). What is emotional intelligence? In P. Salovey & D. Sluyter (Eds.), *Emotional development and emotional intelligence: Implications for educators* (pp. 3–31). Basic Books.

McFerran, K. S. (2000). From the mouths of babes: The response of six younger bereaved teenagers to the experience of psychodynamic group music therapy. *Australian Journal of Music Therapy, 11*, 3–22.

McFerran, K. S. (2016). Contextualising the relationship between music, emotions and the wellbeing of young people: A Critical Interpretive Synthesis. *Musicae Scientiae, 20*(1), 103–121. https://doi.org/10.1177/1029864915626968

McFerran, K. S. (2020). Adolescents and music therapy: Contextualized recommendations for research and practice. *Music Therapy Perspectives, 38*(1), 80–88. https://doi.org/10.1093/mtp/miz014

McFerran, K. S., & Saarikallio, S. (2013). Depending on music to make me feel better: Being conscious of responsibility when appropriating the power of music. *The Arts in Psychotherapy, 41*(1), 89–97. https://doi.org/10.1016/j.aip.2013.11.007

McFerran, K. S., Hense, C., Koike, A., & Rickwood, D. (2018). Intentional music use to reduce psychological distress in adolescents accessing primary mental health care. *Clinical Child Psychology and Psychiatry, 23*(4). 567–581, first published online. https://doi.org/10.1177/1359104518767231

McFerran, K., Derrington, P., & Saarikallio, S. (Eds.). (2019). *Handbook of music, adolescents, and wellbeing.* Oxford University Press.

Miranda, D. (2013). The role of music in adolescent development: Much more than the same old song. *International Journal of Adolescence and Youth, 18*(1), 5–22. https://doi.org/10.1080/02673843.2011.650182

Miranda, D. (2019). Personality traits and music in adolescence. In K. McFerran, P. Derrington, & S. Saarikallio (Eds.), *Handbook of music, adolescents, and wellbeing* (pp. 99–108). Oxford University Press.

Newen, A., de Bruin, L., & Gallagher, S. (2018). 4E cognition: Historical roots, key concepts, and central issues. In A. Newen, L. de Bruin, & S. Gallagher (Eds.), *The Oxford handbook of 4E cognition* (pp. 3–18). Oxford University Press.

North, A. C., Hargreaves, D. J., & O'Neill, S. A. (2000). The importance of music to adolescents. *British Journal of Educational Psychology, 70*, 255–272.

North, A. C., & Hargreaves, D. J. (2008). *The social and applied psychology of music.* Oxford University Press.

Nuttall, P. (2009). Insiders, regulars and tourists: Exploring selves and music consumption in adolescence. *Journal of Consumer Behaviour, 8*(4), 211–221.

Pluretti, R., & Bobkowski, P. S. (2019). Social media, adolescent developmental tasks and music. In K. McFerran, P. Derrington, & S. Saarikallio (Eds.), *Handbook of music, adolescents, and wellbeing* (pp. 207–216). Oxford University Press.

Rickwood, D. J., Telford, N., Mazzer, K., Parker, A., Tanti, C. P., & McGorry, P. D. (2015a). Changes in psychological distress and psychosocial functioning in young people visiting headspace centres for mental health problems. *Medical Journal of Australia, 202*, 537–542. https://doi.org/10.5694/mja14.01696

Rolvsjord, R. (2006). Therapy as empowerment: Clinical and political implications of empowerment philosophy in mental health practises of music therapy. *Voices: A World Forum for Music Therapy, 6*(3). https://doi.org/10.15845/voices.v6i3.283

Rolvsjord, R. (2010). *Resource oriented music therapy.* Barcelona Publishers.

Saarikallio, S. (2018, March). Re-thinking the paradox as catalyzed processing: Enjoyment of sadness in music as facilitated emotional processing [Comment on 'An integrative review of the enjoyment of sadness associated with music' by T. Eerola, J. K. Vuoskoski, H. R. Peltola, V. Putkinen, & K. Schäfer (2018)]. *Physics of Life Review*, 25, 100–121.

Saarikallio, S. (2019a). Access-awareness-agency (AAA) model of music-based social-emotional competence (MuSEC). *Music and Science*, 2, 1–16

Saarikallio, S. (2019b). Music as a resource for agency and empowerment in identity construction. In K. McFerran, P. Derrington, & S. Saarikallio (Eds.), *Handbook of music, adolescents, and wellbeing* (pp. 89–98). Oxford University Press.

Saarikallio, S. (2019c). Music. In S. Hupp & J. Jewell (Eds.), *The encyclopedia of child and adolescent development*. John Wiley & Sons. https://doi.org/10.1002/9781119171492

Saarikallio, S., & Erkkilä, J. (2007). The role of music in adolescents' mood regulation. *Psychology of Music*, 35(1), 88–109.

Saarikallio, S., Gold, C., & McFerran, K. (2015). Development and validation of the Healthy-Unhealthy Music Scale (HUMS). *Child and Adolescent Mental Health*, 20(4), 210–217.

Scrine, E. (2019). Reframing inclusivity: The importance of exploring gender and sexuality in music therapy with all young people. In K. McFerran, P. Derrington, & S. Saarikallio (Eds.), *Handbook of music, adolescents, and wellbeing* (pp. 151–161). Oxford University Press.

Schwartz, S. J., Donnellan, M. B., Ravert, R. D., Luyck, K., & Zamboanga, B. L. (2013). Identity development, personality, and well-being in adolescence and emerging adulthood: Theory, research, and recent advances. In R. M. Lerner, M. A. Easterbrooks, J. Mistry, & I. B. Weiner (Eds.), *Handbook of psychology* (2nd ed., pp. 339–364). John Wiley & Sons.

Stern, D. N. (1999). Vitality contours: The temporal contour of feelings as a basic unit for constructing the infant's social experience. In P. Rochat (Ed.), *Early social cognition: Understanding others in the first months of life* (pp. 67–80). Psychology Press.

Thomas, L. A., De Bellis, M. D., Graham, R., & La Bar, K. S. (2007). Development of emotional facial recognition in late childhood and adolescence. *Developmental Science*, 10, 547–558.

Trevarthen, C., & Aitken, K. J. (2001). Infant intersubjectivity: Research, theory, and clinical applications. *The Journal of Child Psychology and Psychiatry and Allied Disciplines*, 42(1), 3–48.

Van Beveren, M. L., Goossens, L., Volkaert, B., Grassmann, C., Wante, L., Vandeweghe, L., Verbeken, S., & Braet, C. (2019). How do I feel right now? Emotional awareness, emotion regulation, and depressive symptoms in youth. *European Child & Adolescent Psychiatry*, 28, 389–398.https://doi.org/10.1007/s00787-018-1203-3

Vetter, N. C., Drauschke, M., Thieme, J., & Altgassen, M. (2018). Adolescent basic facial emotion recognition is not influenced by puberty or own-age bias. *Frontiers in Psychology*, 9, Article 956. https://doi.org/10.3389/fpsyg.2018.00956

Viega, M. (2019). Globalizing adolescence: Digital music cultures and music therapy. In K. McFerran, P. Derrington, & S. Saarikallio (Eds.), *Handbook of music, adolescents, and wellbeing* (pp. 217–224). Oxford University Press.

Ward, D., & Stapleton, M. (2012). Es are good: Cognition as enacted, embodied, embedded, affective and extended. In F. Paglieri (Ed.), *Consciousness in interaction: The role of the natural and social context in shaping consciousness* (pp. 86–89) [e-book version]. John Benjamins Publishing. http://ebookcentral.proquest.com

Westerlund, H., Partti, H., & Karlsen, S. (2017). Identity formation and agency in the diverse music classroom. In R. MacDonald, D. Hargreaves, & D. Miell (Eds.), *Handbook of musical identities* (pp. 493–509). Oxford University Press.

World Health Organization. (2020a). *Adolescent health*. https://www.who.int/health-topics/adolescent-health#tab=tab_1

World Health Organization. (2020b). *Adolescent mental health*. https://www.who.int/news-room/fact-sheets/detail/adolescent-mental-health

Wölfl, A. (2019). Music and violence: Working with youth to prevent violence. In K. McFerran, P. Derrington, & S. Saarikallio (Eds.), *Handbook of music, adolescents, and wellbeing* (pp. 75–86). Oxford University Press.

Zeman, J., Cassano, M., Perry-Parrish, C., & Stegall, S. (2006). Emotion regulation in children and adolescents. *Journal of Developmental & Behavioral Pediatrics, 27*(2), 155–168.

4
Musical care in adulthood

Sounding our way through the landscape

Simon Procter and Tia DeNora

Introduction: Age and age-bands are social products

This chapter addresses the intersection of two broad ideas: musical care (complementary understandings of which are outlined elsewhere in this volume) and adulthood itself, understood as a cultural construction within the larger construct of the 'life course', and therefore also as a social role and subject to expectations, obligations, and—not infrequently—socially generated forms of physical and mental stress.

Normative categories of age, the life course, and ageing are, for all practical purposes, *real* because they are routinely enacted. They are produced and performed and are therefore constructions (Holstein & Gubrium, 2007). Even biological capacities and states may be understood as the product of real-time situated practices and sociocultural-technical milieux (Langer, 2009). The case of adulthood is, arguably, especially interesting because so much of the 'work' involved in becoming and remaining 'an adult' is less visible than it is in other life course stages (such as childhood, adolescence, and old age).

If, as Hammack & Toolis (2014) suggest, adulthood is best conceived as a cultural discourse, then we need to consider how music gets into and shapes the content of age-banded realities. How is music part of the negotiation and achievement of adulthood? How is musical self-care part of the set of practices required for 'being an adult'? And how are age-linked forms of care and self-care using music part of how adulthood itself is produced and sustained?

Becoming, and remaining, an 'adult'

Adulthood is often considered to be the stage at which we are at our zenith. In adulthood, the story goes, we are no longer children, dependent on our caregivers. Nor are we adolescents struggling to claim an identity in the world. We have not yet succumbed to the various deteriorations of old age that may once again render us dependent on others and economically unproductive. As adults, we are expected to be

Simon Procter and Tia DeNora, *Musical care in adulthood* In: *Collaborative Insights*. Edited by: Neta Spiro and Katie Rose M. Sanfilippo, Oxford University Press. © Oxford University Press 2022. DOI: 10.1093/oso/9780197535011.003.0005 self-assured, capable, resilient, and healthy human units. Adulthood as a life stage is thus assumed to be both clear (in terms of when we are adults) and stable. Each of these assumptions bears brief examination at the outset.

The onset of adulthood is legally significant because it confers legal responsibility and, in theory at least, full rights as a citizen—although these are clearly unequally distributed in practice—and is usually legally determined according to chronological age. In the absence of chronological documentation, proxy biological measures, including dental maturity, are commonly used to assign such status, although even this assigning is done with geographical and cultural caveats (e.g., Zelic et al., 2016). In neither sociological nor psychological terms, however, can the onset of adulthood be pinned to a date on the calendar: neither is its nature universally agreed upon.

Pilcher et al. (2003) and Blatterer (2007) bemoan their fellow sociologists' neglect of adulthood, despite its being 'the unarticulated background to a majority of social enquiries' (Blatterer, 2007, p. 771), contrasting this more sociological perspective with psychology's definitional tendency. Nevertheless, there is a long-standing interdisciplinary dissatisfaction with the prevailing 'taken for granted' nature of adulthood in particular focusing on the transition from childhood or adolescence to adulthood. Blos (1941) describes as 'post-adolescence' the stage inhabited by individuals who seem to be deferring their definitive acceptance of adulthood. Peller (1946) points out its dialectical nature, with the anticipation of adulthood framing experiences of childhood just as childhood experiences shape adulthood. More recently there have been multidisciplinary attempts to redescribe the transition, with many psychologists embracing Arnett's call for the recognition of a phase of 'emerging adulthood' (Armett, 2004).

Neither is adulthood static. Life-affecting conditions continue into (and develop within) adulthood, and life-changing events can occur at any time. When adults encounter 'troubles' there are, of course, a range of people who put themselves forward to help get them back 'on track'—counsellors, psychiatrists, family therapists, spiritual leaders, doctors, and New Age providers of everything from horoscopes to aromatherapy. And then there is music.

The role of music in the approach to adulthood has been considered (e.g., by Agbo-Quaye & Robertson, 2010), as have how adults' tastes, identities, and social habits may shift as their circumstances and experiences change (Bonneville-Roussy et al., 2013). Adults may become parents (as discussed in the Musical care in infancy chapter) or find themselves carers for others. And whereas medicine traditionally views people as discrete units, in practice we are interlinked by relationships, by membership of overlapping communities, circumstantial or otherwise, and by the impact on us of broader social, political, and economic shifts. Where these factors aid adults in their flourishing they are generally ignored. But sometimes their negative effects can be crippling, as in the cases of deprivation, discrimination, persecution, and war.

Even in less extreme circumstances, adulthood is rarely likely to be experienced as a smooth plateau between adolescence and old age. Life course studies emphasize how development occurs throughout life: most people are able to give accounts of the vicissitudes encountered along the trajectory of adulthood. After accidental death, suicide is the most common cause of death in young men worldwide (Pitman et al., 2012). The levels of mental illness diagnosed in Western societies attest to adulthood not being plain sailing for everyone, and this finding is taking into account only in those cases of mental distress which are known to the medical system. We know that many people manage (with varying degrees of success) troubling feelings and experiences without medical help by using self-care—whether they do so alone or via the support of friends and community.

So, while adulthood (whenever it occurs and whatever form it takes) is typically described as the phase of life in which formalized care is least expected to be necessary (although mutual low-level emotional care as part of a mutual relationship is likely to be an aspiration of most adults), the reality of being an adult includes pressure to look as though one were well, coping, and engaging in the public world of work and/or caring for family members. For these reasons, adults often hide vulnerabilities or needs for care until the point where these have become serious, when something goes 'really wrong', and when the person's life trajectory may be seen as markedly deviant from the rhetorical 'norm'. Within this 'all or nothing' continuum of adult wellness, when things go 'really wrong' they may bring on a sense of loss (of normality, of future possibilities, of expected self), not only for the person concerned but also for those to whom they are connected, for whom they are responsible, and for whom they care. How, then, do, and can, 'adults' manage their well-being so as to remain functioning 'adults'? Why, within the reality of adulthood, is it important to consider the often-tacit, often-hidden forms of self-care that keep adults 'adult'? And finally, how does consideration of self-care and musical care in daily life enrich music therapeutic approaches to adulthood and its various distresses?

Musical care within adulthood: A mapping of the chapter

What kinds of care occur within adulthood? We approach this question from dual perspectives—music therapy and cultural sociology. The literatures emanating from nursing, care work, and care institutions tend to focus on professionalized 'caregiving' (which is frequently also commercial and linked to the burgeoning care industry) or familial care roles, configuring care as a required response to an often-medicalized situation.

However, in daily life, care and self-care are routinely needed by everyone (DeNora, 2000; Skånland, 2013). Musical care takes place in lay form (building on folk knowledge and everyday expertise) as well as in more organized or professionalized forms such as music therapy. This chapter therefore considers four aspects of musical care— that associated with self-care, that associated with familial or emotional ties, that which is associated with industrialized and commercialized provision, and finally 'music therapy' and related specifically musical forms of service provision, whether these are professionalized or not. In practice, these aspects overlap considerably, and we distinguish between them here simply in order to highlight different perspectives and angles.

We propose a conception of musical care within adulthood as a potential opening up of cultural, aesthetic, and interpersonal opportunities for action (Ruud, 2008), mutually crafted, with implications for all concerned (not just the 'carer'). Musical care can be considered a means of constructing (and rescuing) emergent identity amidst the challenges of adulthood. This point is considered within the context of biographical trajectory (e.g., Hooper & Procter, 2013) and has potential to subvert the unidirectionality commonly ascribed to medicalized or industrialized notions of care that took shape during the 20th century in relation to political economies of health—medicine for profit, medical insurance, and the very notion of a specialist province of 'health care'.

Musical self-care: Music as a technology of the self

Much self-care goes unreported, even unnoticed, even by those engaging in their own self-care. It is therefore unsurprising that musical self-care remains largely unexamined. Although Western ethnomusicology has gone to 'faraway lands', observing how people make use of music and musical activity for apparently non-musical reasons (healing rituals, for example), this same degree of observational learning is applied far less within the same Western societies that have sent out those ethnomusicologists (Koen, 2012). In part this avoidance is a legacy of music's status as an autonomous 'art' form in Western societies, but it may also reflect the dominance of medical models of health and illness within Western cultures. Nevertheless, the music sociology literature offers many accounts not only of ways in which people make music, but also of ways in which they use music to configure their experiences of themselves and of the (inherently social) world around them (DeNora, 2003). Batt-Rawden et al. (2005) show how music listening as a lay or folk healing practice can enhance well-being and 'wellness' for people living with long-term illnesses and diseases by offering resources for recovery and quality of life. This finding flags up the fuzzy nature of care, and of the associated notions of health and well-being. The boundary between someone doing something to be happy, or entertained/distracted, and doing something to look after themselves is not clear: indeed, these things necessarily overlap. Thus, we need to attend to a broad range of musical practices that people report engaging in, even if these are not specifically portrayed as forms of self-care.

Another issue that may obscure our view of musical self-care is the professionalization of music therapy and the associated assumption that a trained professional is required to administer treatment to a client if musical care of some sort is to happen. Yet many people speak readily about how 'music is my therapy', whether this is by (seemingly) *passive* listening to music, or by *active* participation in music-making.

The terms passive and active are, of course, overly simplistic. In daily life for many people, private 'listening' to music is also the way that active music-making happens, whether this takes the form of singing in the shower or copying the dance routines associated with particular songs. For people who consider themselves musicians, in private is generally where they do their backstage musical work—spending time with their instrument, learning to do new things or to play new material. All of these forms of musical engagement can be understood as 'self work'. An interdisciplinary area of study that has focused attention on such work to varying degrees is the 'everyday life' perspective. In relation to music this has spread from being a primarily sociological concern (e.g., DeNora, 2000) to now also being a significant category of work within music psychology (Sloboda, 2010).

DeNora (1999) outlines music's role as a 'technology of the self', providing a 'scaffolding for self-constitution' and making possible multiple forms of 'mundane self-care and self-regulation' (2007, p. 277). Examples of this role include people's use of music as a means of emotional self-regulation, as also discussed in the context of the Musical care in adolescence chapter, of preparing themselves for a social task or event, and of programming their music listening in ways that build on their awareness of certain musics having certain 'effects' on them. In many cases of musical self-care, it is possible to see how adults' uses of music to 'gear up' or 'calm down' are linked to adult responsibilities and to things that they might not always 'want' to do, such as undertaking paid work. Indeed, music's role as a technology of the 'worker-self' is an important part of adult musical engagement, both outside the workplace and within it. Music motivates and regulates and is used to pass the time in otherwise boring or challenging work environments (Korczynski et al., 2013).

In this sense, the musical care of self is as much about engaging in the forms of 'emotional labour' associated with occupational roles and tasks (Hochschild, 1983) as it is about self-actualization or well-being. The care of self is part of the 'work' that adults do to be able to function in 'adult' roles and to complete tasks that they might prefer to avoid. That care also involves, at times, forms of musical 'time travelling' when adults listen to the music of their youth, becoming, virtually and for a short period of time, young again (DeNora, 2019). Skånland (2013) has observed how recent developments in portable music players has enabled this conscious affect regulation to happen not just in private but also beyond the home.

How music 'helps' in all of these examples seems to have to do with a combination of musical characteristics of the music itself, personal and generic associations, and the activities and situations that are framing the music. As DeNora makes clear, 'music's affordances are found in and through active practices of listening or otherwise appropriating music' (2007, p. 278). A celebrated example of this notion is provided by Gomart & Hennion (1999), who draw parallels between the intricate ways in which people prepare themselves for listening to music so that its full effects can be experienced and the ways in which drug users do the same in relation to taking drugs. Work is required for the affordances of music to be appropriated. In this way people actively strive to 'collude in their own subjection to musical/material "control"' (DeNora, 2007, p. 278).

Many self-care practices that are not specifically musical nevertheless have musical dimensions to them—e.g., attendance at aerobics classes, where tutors will choose music that can be experienced as 'helping' attendees to fulfil the requirements of the class (DeNora, 2000). Equally, attendance at communal religious observance may well include active or (apparently) passive involvement in music-making. These forms of music-making may become associated with building and sustaining a sense of membership and identity even when people are not actually there, thus acting as an aspect of care by cementing a sustaining and protective sense of belonging.

Estroff (1995) describes observing a former psychiatric patient singing in her church choir and realizing how choral singing was enabling much of what rehabilitation aims for in an authentic and sustainable way. Choirs can be social and supportive of identity, offering people a very different experience of themselves and their singing. A growing literature addresses potential benefits of singing per se as well as social singing in choirs and other vocal groups. (e.g., Clift, 2012), as discussed in the Musical care in older adulthood chapter. Lamont et al. (2018) highlight social relationships, meaning, and accomplishment as ways in which older people find choral participation beneficial for their well-being, also emphasizing the need for sustainable, skilled musical leadership. A large-scale questionnaire-based study across the adult age ranges (Moss et al., 2018) reports multiple benefits with significant gender variations. The popularity of this research area is demonstrated by the recent publication of an 'Agenda for Best Practice Research on Group Singing, Health, and Well-Being' (Dingle et al., 2019). There is less work on non-choir social situations wherein non-older adults sing or otherwise make music together: e.g., brass bands (Williamson & Bonshor, 2019).

However, not all everyday uses of music can be seen as self-care. As highlighted in the Musical care in adolescence chapter, McFerran and Saarikallio (2014) report that young people struggling with their mental health may use music for rumination and self-isolation. Although a retreat into music can make a person feel better, the fact that they are removing themselves—and becoming isolated—from precisely the environments they find disturbing leads to a further distancing from the skills and practices that it would take to engage with, and perhaps surmount, the difficulties posed by the social worlds that they need to navigate and inhabit. So too for those who work in musical industries, music can become noxious because of the relentless emphasis on competition and profit (Gross & Musgrave, 2016).

Musical care associated with familial or emotional ties

We now turn our attention towards the idea of one person caring for another. We will start with the most natural version of this: the intuitive care that most commonly takes place within families or established personal relationships.

Much of the care associated with emotional or familial ties happens behind closed doors and therefore is largely inaccessible to observation: hence its sparse examination in the literature (with some exceptions: e.g., Custodero, 2009). Much of this care is lay activity in the sense that carers have not been specifically trained to deliver care in any form (let alone musical care): they are unlikely to consider themselves to be expert carers, never mind musical carers.

The most researched example is the musical care of infants by their parents (see the Musical care in infancy chapter for examples). An entire subdiscipline of psychology has grown out of detailed observation of such interactions, which are not at all one-way and are characterized by the use of identifiable musical elements such as rhythm, timing, melodic phrase, and turn-taking (Trevarthen, 2002) even when the parents are not thinking about what they are doing in musical terms. This is a significant caregiving experience for the adults concerned because (although the physical task of caring falls to the adult) the benefits are demonstrably experienced also by the adult (Fancourt & Perkins, 2017).

Less open to scrutiny (and less comfortable to contemplate having to experience) is the position that many adults find themselves in, of becoming de facto carers for other adults. These may be their grown-up children, siblings, or partners who have learning disabilities or who have suffered injury, illness, or trauma, whether in adulthood or in earlier life. Or these may be their parents who have developed dementia or physical incapacities (as will be discussed in the next chapter, on Musical care in older adulthood. Most find themselves in this role through force of circumstance, and where this becomes a long-term or permanent role it is likely to be accompanied by a significant interruption of life plans accompanied by substantial emotional upheaval. Another consequence of this unforeseen situation may be the significant economic impact of having to give up a job, as well as the accompanying loss of independence and the ability to engage in previously shared pleasurable activities.

Family carers usually come to caring for a loved one with a background of their relationship with that person. This is significant in musical terms, because music plays a significant role within intimate and family relationships. Songs and other music carry significance in ways that may be known only to those two people, or to their family. Thus, music becomes a means of continuing a prior relationship of intimacy across the rupture of a life-changing event that may in other respects appear to change dramatically the nature of the relationship. Equally, it may sustain an intimate dimension to a lifelong caring relationship (e.g., of a parent with a profoundly disabled adult son or daughter). It mediates more usual considerations of age appropriacy and eases situations that might otherwise be unbearable. It can also function as a shortcut in expression of the relationship: for example, an elderly parent singing a lullaby to their learning-disabled adult child might transport them both to an easier phase of their relationship many years ago without any need for words. The paucity of research in this area is attributable to the difficulties in accessing such intimate moments of everyday life; nevertheless, this is a field for sensitive future work.

Musical dimensions of industrialized and commercialized provision of care

Here we turn our attention to musical interactions that may occur within situations in which people are paid to care for other adults. This category includes care workers as well as nursing and care management roles.

Some areas of paid care work are portrayed as low skilled and therefore undeserving of financial rewards, with many positions being minimally paid (England et al., 2002; Palmer & Eveline, 2012). The commercialized provision of care in the form of the burgeoning 'care industry' is leveraged by the financially powerful in order to further advantage their position (McKee & Stuckler, 2012). When training is provided it tends to consist of basic units that protect the care company from prosecution. There is little attention to the craft of care work, but even a cursory examination of care work in action reveals care workers drawing on a range of skills, understandings, aptitudes, and experience, whether or not these are made explicit, and regardless of their economic value. These are craft skills, and for the purposes of this chapter we will focus on how musical craft skills (whether intentional or not) can be observed to contribute to people's experience of care environments.

As poorly paid and supposedly 'low-skilled' work, paid care roles in Western nations are frequently performed (with great skill) by migrant workers (Nordberg, 2016; Williams, 2012): sometimes this situation seems to be associated with a greater readiness to use music, in particular to sing and dance with the people they are caring for. Of all forms of music-making, these are the most immediately engaging for many people because of their innate physicality and the musical companionship on offer. The use of singing or dancing may not originate as a conscious act of caring for another: it may be a means of attending to one's own identity in an unappreciative environment, or of coping with the hard, repetitive physical work that is central to much 'care' work. But even in such cases, it becomes a means of presentation of self in the workplace (Goffman, 1959), and as such it also becomes another way in which connection can occur between carer and the person they are caring for.

Many able carers demonstrate considerable, although often unconscious, skill in the musical engagement of, motivation of, and attending to people who often find such engagement challenging because they need more time, or because trust is not easy. A skilled carer can draw on musical structure in their approach to a service user in a way that turns the repetition and predictability of songs or dances into repeated and predictable opportunities for connection. Rather than singing an entire song or doing an entire dance, they may use elements of these with real purpose to engage someone, to attend to them, and to ease the performance of required tasks such as washing or brushing teeth (as parents might instinctively do with their own young children). Such experiences lead over time to a sense of connection and engagement, thanks both to the characteristics of the musical elements used, and also to the work (of framing the encounters) being put in by the carer.

This is not music miraculously making someone feel cared for—rather, the making of music in the form of singing and/or dancing takes place as part of a broader process of care. This is ostensibly performed by one person (who is paid) for another person (who is in need), but in fact there is often once again a degree of mutuality about this relationship in that the carer is likely to experience the response of the 'cared for' person as a kind of personal connection, or at the very least something different from habitual behaviours that may sometimes be very challenging and dispiriting. In this way the use of music is mediated by the care situation but also acts upon the situation. Such situational craft skills are worthy of careful examination—a rare example, albeit from the world of dementia care, is provided by Wood (2020).

Much has been written in studies of care work and nursing about emotional labour (Hochschild, 1983; Huynh et al., 2008; Theodosius, 2008)—the often-hidden requirements of people to manage their feelings in certain ways in order to be able to do a job. The use of singing and dancing in care work by supposedly non-musician staff could be considered a means of coping with the emotional demands of working with vulnerable and often demanding people. Rather than having to respond in a directly personal or emotional manner, a musical presentation of self to the other can be considered to offer a means of containing anxieties and vulnerabilities (on both sides) within the structure and potential certainties of musical interaction.

In addition to these 'naturally occurring' musical dimensions of industrialized care work, there is also a growing focus within the nursing literature on the intentional use of music within such care environments for the achievement of certain goals. A recent mapping study suggests that nurses' use of (mostly receptive) music interventions is more widespread than might be imagined (Ciğerci et al., 2019) and engagement in music has been identified (amongst many other possibilities) as an effective self-care strategy for nurses (Kravits et al, 2010).

Specific musical care provision in the form of music therapy and associated professionalized and non-professionalized activities

Finally, we turn our attention to the specific provision of musical services to adults needing care. We use the term 'musical services' here to bracket formats like performance, workshop, or session, each of which carries varying implications and may be used by different groups of musicians, including music therapists, community musicians, and music and health practitioners.

In some places, including the United Kingdom, Austria, and some parts of the United States, statutory regulation has restricted the use of the term 'music therapy', with non-therapist practitioners using workaround terms such as 'therapeutic music' or 'music for health'. For our purposes here we will simply consider together the various ways in which musicians set out to offer services to adults in need of care, especially in formalized settings such as care homes, hospitals, and hospices.

Intentional musical provision gets delivered in a range of formats. Some of these are fundamentally social in the sense that they draw upon music's capacity to promote social interaction and offer new experiences of self in relation to other. They also have the capacity to offer something ecological to the setting (which in care contexts might mean a home, a care home, a hospice, or a day centre) by affecting the atmosphere of the place with consequences for quality of life (Batt-Rawden & Storlien, 2019). Furthermore, musical groups can become improvised contexts of care wherein service users are enabled to engage in mutual care in ways that are less obvious or stigmatizing than might be possible elsewhere.

A common social format is that of a choir or singing group. In some cases, the focus is on working towards performance, and in others simply on the group's experience of singing together or of working on material together. Sometimes there is a specific agenda of promoting wider social interaction, with the music-making *being* the wider social interaction. Some mental health organizations support or set up choirs on the basis of principles of social inclusion (Plumb & Stickley, 2017).

Another social opportunity for musical collaboration is the band. For many adults, this format accords more closely with their own cultural values and musical aspirations than singing in a choir, and it also has the advantage of offering distinct roles (drummer, guitarist, keyboard player, etc.) that people can invest in over time as they gain skills and get to know one another better. This kind of work is widely reported in prisons (e.g., Hjørnevik & Waage, 2019)—perhaps not traditionally seen as a care environment, but one where adults are vulnerable and their mental health is at risk. Being a band member rather than a 'client' offers service users a greater degree of responsibility and autonomy. Bands can even outlive their members' statuses as service users and provide a musical pathway into a healthy, safe lifestyle beyond the initial care (or incarceration) context (e.g., Tuastad & Stige, 2018).

Part of any care relationship is 'how' one person works to be with others, and how this availability can be conveyed perceptibly. Musically, this role is about accompaniment. Thus, for many musicians working in care environments the initial way of 'meeting' someone is to accompany them musically. Doing so means hearing all that they have to offer as music and responding to this—not initially in order to change it but rather to make clear that the service user's role is the solo part and the musician's part merely the accompaniment. This is a real skill and could be described as 'extreme accompaniment',[1] because what is being offered in the first place is not necessarily intended as music. It requires acute listening and musical imagination as well as a range of musical techniques in order to be able to tailor one's music to whatever is being offered (Ansdell, 1995).

A step on from accompaniment is the notion of musical companionship (Ansdell & Pavlicevic, 2005), in which an experience of togetherness arises from shared

[1] We are grateful to Rachel Verney for this term.

music-making. In music therapy circles this is often linked to the idea of a working alliance or therapeutic relationship. This may be conceived of as a personal companionship, or it may be more of an 'in this moment, in this music' experience. Such companionship then opens up the possibilities of shared work featuring challenge, change, and development (e.g., Aigen, 1998).

Songwriting can be a powerful means of engaging people in a collaborative (and often iterative) process that yields something distinctively theirs: this approach is employed across a wide range of settings and 'client groups', including neurorehabilitation and mental health services. In the adult care system, individuality is often compromised and the expression of identity that can happen in a song is invaluable, especially if this outcome can be coupled with appropriate opportunities for performance, whether within the care environment or beyond. Songwriting is a recurring element of the literature within both music therapy (Aasgaard & Ærø 2016; Baker, 2015; Edgerton, 1990), and community music (e.g., Higgins, 2012; Kumm, 2013; MacDonald, 2013).

For some service users, especially within mental health provision, skilled musical services offer an opportunity to rediscover earlier connections with music, or to discover ways of using music in everyday life that help to sustain health (i.e., the use of music as self-care, as discussed previously). It is common to hear stories of how involvement in music was lost at the time of a life crisis: an important part of the work of a musician in such contexts can be helping to reconnect people with music. For examples see Hooper & Procter (2013) and Ansdell & DeNora (2016).

Gathering the musical scenes together

At the heart of all these examples of musical care work in adulthood is the intertwinedness of people, music, social role, and social situation. Music is never an autonomous intervention. It needs people to engage in careful work if it is to do its job of offering opportunities for action—being, doing, feeling, and relating. These in turn impact on the situation and the people engaging in it. Music is not a magic bullet or stimulus and does not work like a drug; music offers culturally learned ways of being—alone and with others. In relation to adult care, music offers, for example, ways to sustain one's role, to hold on to the energy and motivation to care for others. It offers a medium with which to engage in that care for others. It offers resources for reconnecting with others when cognitive capacities deteriorate. And it offers a medium with which to recover—self, mental orientation, and outlook, whether through music's use as a kind of proto-social capital that primes social bonding and network development (Procter, 2011) or as a means of self-development or transferrable skill, as discussed previously. Much of what music offers arises from people's musical histories and identities, in ways that illuminate childhood musical practices as legacy resources for adulthood and beyond. It is an exercising of expertise, of experiencing life, and of developing identity that is often undervalued, particularly in the context of clinical attitudes to health and well-being (DeNora, 2013). Identity studies is an interdisciplinary area both in general (e.g., du Gay et al., 2000) and in relation to music (e.g., MacDonald et al., 2017): the intertwining of musical biography and musical identity remains a key area of work at both individual and social levels.

Directions for future research

Care is frequently seen as the poor relation of intervention or treatment. Research focusing on treatment tends to attract more funding and prestige than research focusing on care. Yet, as we hope we have shown in this chapter, care is a complex, relational, intersubjective, and multifaceted aspect of human interaction that is not needed only at moments of obvious crisis or at the beginning and end of life. It demands our attention as researchers because it challenges many of our assumptions about life. It speaks of our vulnerabilities and frailties as human beings, of our interdependence and of our potential neediness. But most of all care is remarkable for its ubiquity and necessity. It is for many people an unchosen life's work, and music is a routinely used means of getting that work done that is too often neglected by research.

Much medical-style research assumes music to be a discrete 'intervention' that can be applied to an identified problem in order to produce a measurable improvement, thus neglecting the social complexity of what happens within mundane practices of care as well as the socio-musical expertise contributed by supposed 'recipients' of care.

As researchers, we need to do more to learn more about the nature of musical engagement as it gets deployed in everyday care: the realm of adulthood is often the place where this kind of care is at its most routine and most invisible. The notion of the 'everyday' has become somewhat 'smoothed over' in the literature, as though 'everyday' referred only to unproblematic and unremarkable aspects of life. Like the common uses of adulthood, it brings with it a sense of 'nothing interesting to see here'. Yet, for many adults, difficulty, pain, impairment, isolation, despair, depression, and grief are all part of 'everyday life'. Everyday life is complex, not straightforward: it is characterized by vicissitudes, and any examination of it needs to examine also the ways people act in order to cope with these vicissitudes—for themselves as well as for and with one another. It is clear that some of these ways are inherently musical, even when people are not thinking about what they do as 'making music'. We need to avoid the peculiarly Western trap of examining 'music' as something set apart from other aspects of everyday life (Small, 1998). Music doesn't just happen in predetermined places or at predetermined times: it weaves like a thread through so much of what we do that is personal, social, and interactional. Like a thread it is often given little attention because it is perceived as purely decorative when in fact it is holding things together: indeed, by holding things together, it becomes the things themselves. People sometimes talk of their life being held together by music: this isn't just a lazy expression (Ansdell & DeNora, 2016).

Hence, we are calling for future research to attend to the care work of music and the musical work of care in real, naturally occurring situations, whether these feature the work of music therapists or community musicians, the possibly unthinkingly musical work of people who care for others (whether professionally or familially), and also the work that people do to help themselves cope, survive, and thrive. We need to be much more sensitive to where and when musical care occurs—not simply inspecting it where it is pre-planned. This means a musical sensitivity to mundane social interaction as well as attention to unfolding musical detail within those events.

In theoretical terms, much contemporary work in the area of how people use music to get things done (or equally how music helps people to get things done) draws on the idea of affordance and appropriation. This idea was first offered by Gibson (1958) but has been specifically applied to the use of music within everyday life by DeNora (2000) and Clarke (2005). The notion of 'musical event' (DeNora, 2003; DeNora & Ansdell, 2017) has been developed as an analytic tool to help actualize this theoretical work in the realization of detailed observational research. It seeks to trace closely how people's past experiences and associations are drawn into their real-time engagement with music and then drawn out and on into subsequent acts and experiences. So, for example, we may bring to the listening/performing event prior associations, memories, or tastes. We then take away new memories and new associations and connections with that music and the situation of engagement with music. This simple analytic device can be used for musical engagement in any setting and is well suited to the topic of musical care.

A strong heritage of ethnographic and ethnomusicological work attends to the minutiae of music as it occurs in particular social situations. This heritage now needs to be extended to include a detailed focus on how music as care gets achieved in practice (focusing not only on professionalized practice but also on lay expertise), on how music is understood as a means of care, and on the role of mutuality in music as care. All this then needs to be set alongside work that focuses more medically on the 'effects' of music used in various situations. These are necessarily interdisciplinary concerns, and greater collaboration is needed to generate an understanding of the role of musical care in adulthood, an understanding that is not only broader in view but also more accessible in applicability.

References

Aasgaard, T., & Ærø, S. (2016). Songwriting techniques in music therapy practice. In J. Edwards (Ed.), *The Oxford handbook of music therapy* (pp. 644–668). Oxford University Press. https://www.oxfordhandbooks.com/view/10.1093/oxfordhb/9780199639755.001.0001/oxfordhb-9780199639755-e-20

Agbo-Quaye, S., & Robertson, T. (2010). The motorway to adulthood: Music preference as the sex and relationships roadmap. *Sex Education, 10*(4), 359–371.

Aigen, K. (1998). *Paths of development in Nordoff-Robbins music therapy*. Barcelona Publishers.

Ansdell, G. (1995). *Music for life: Aspects of creative music therapy with adult clients*. Jessica Kingsley Publishers.

Ansdell, G., & Pavlicevic, M. (2005). Musical companionship, musical community: Music therapy and the process and value of musical communication. In D. Miell, R. MacDonald, & D. Hargreaves (Eds.), *Musical communication* (pp. 193–213). Oxford University Press.

Ansdell, G., & DeNora, T. (2016). *Musical pathways in recovery: Community music therapy and mental wellbeing*. Routledge.

Arnett, J. J. (2004). *Emerging adulthood: The winding road from the late teens through the twenties*. Oxford University Press.

Baker, F. A. (2015). *Therapeutic songwriting: Developments in theory, methods and practice*. Palgrave Macmillan.

Batt-Rawden, K., DeNora, T., & Ruud, E. (2005). Music listening and empowerment in health promotion: A study of the role and significance of music in everyday life of the long-term ill *Nordic Journal of Music Therapy, 14*(2), 120–136.

Batt-Rawden, K., & Storlien, M. (2019). Systematic use of music as an environmental intervention and quality of care in nursing homes: A qualitative case study in Norway. *Medicines, 6*(1), 12. https://doi.org/10.3390/medicines6010012

Blatterer, H. (2007). Contemporary adulthood: Reconceptualizing an uncontested category. *Current Sociology, 55*(6), 771–792.

Blos, P. (1941). *The adolescent personality: A study of individual behavior for the commission on secondary school curriculum of the Progressive Education Association*. Appleton-Century.

Bonneville-Roussy, A., Rentfrow, P. J., Xu, M. K., & Potter, J. (2013). Music through the ages: Trends in musical engagement and preferences from adolescence through middle adulthood. *Journal of Personality and Social Psychology, 105*(4), 703–717.

Ciğerci, Y., Kısacık, Ö., Özyürek, P., & Çevik, C. (2019). Nursing music intervention: A systematic mapping study. *Complementary Therapies in Clinical Practice, 35*, 109–120.

Clarke, E. (2005). *Ways of listening: An ecological approach to the perception of musical meaning*. Oxford University Press.

Clift, S. (2012). Singing, wellbeing, and health. In R. A. R. MacDonald, G. Kreutz, & L. Mitchell (Eds.), *Music, health, and wellbeing* (pp. 113–124). Oxford University Press.

Custodero, L. (2009). Musical portraits, musical pathways: Stories of meaning making in the lives of six families. In J. Kerchner & C. Abril (Eds.), *Musical experience in our lives: The things we learn and meanings we make* (pp. 77–92). Rowman and Littlefield.

DeNora, T. (1999) Music as a technology of the self. *Poetics, 27*(1), 31–56.

DeNora, T. (2000). *Music in everyday life*. Cambridge University Press.

DeNora, T (2003). *After Adorno: Rethinking music sociology*. Cambridge University Press.

DeNora, T. (2007) Health and music in everyday life: A theory of practice. *Psyke & Logos, 28*(1), 271–287.

DeNora, T. (2013). *Music asylums: Wellbeing through music in everyday life*. Ashgate.

DeNora, T. (2019). 'Forever piping songs forever new': The musical teenager and the musical inner teenager across the life course. In K. McFerran, P. Derrington, & S. Saarikallio (Eds.), *Handbook of music, adolescents, and wellbeing* (pp. 119–126). Oxford University Press.

DeNora, T., & Ansdell, G. (2017). Music in action: Tinkering, testing and tracing over time. *Qualitative Research, 17*(2), 231–245.

Dingle, G. A., Clift, S., Finn, S., Gilbert, R., Groarke, J. M., Irons, J. Y., Bartoli, A. J., Lamont, A., Launay, J., Martin, E. S., Moss, H., Sanfilippo, K. R., Shipton, M., Stewart, L., Talbot, S., Tarrant, M., Tip, L., & Williams, E. J. (2019). An agenda for best practice research on group singing, health, and well-being. *Music & Science, 2*, 1–15. https://doi.org/10.1177/2059204319861719

du Gay, P., Evans, J., & Redman, P. (2000). *Identity: A reader*. Sage Publications.

Edgerton, C. D. (1990). Creative group songwriting. *Music Therapy Perspectives, 8*(1), 15–19.

England, P., Budig, M., & Folbre, N. (2002). Wages of virtue: The relative pay of care work. *Social Problems, 49*(4), 455–473.

Estroff, S. E. (1995) Brokenhearted lifetimes: Ethnography, subjectivity and psychosocial rehabilitation. *International Journal of Mental Health, 24*(1), 82–92.

Fancourt, D., & Perkins, R. (2017). Associations between singing to babies and symptoms of postnatal depression, wellbeing, self-esteem and mother-infant bond. *Public Health, 145,* 149–152.

Gibson, J. J. (1958). *The senses considered as perceptual systems.* Houghton Mifflin.

Goffman, E. (1959). *The presentation of self in everyday life.* Doubleday Anchor.

Gomart, E., & Hennion, A. (1999). A sociology of attachment: Music amateurs, drug users. In J. Law & J. Hassard (Eds.), *Actor network theory and after* (pp. 220–247). Blackwell.

Gross, S. A., & Musgrave, G. (2016). *Can music make you sick? Music and depression: A study into the incidence of musicians' mental health. Part 1: Pilot survey report.* MusicTank.

Hammack, P. L., & Toolis, E. (2014). Narrative and the social construction of adulthood. In B. Schiff (Ed.), *Rereading personal narrative and life course: New directions in child and adolescent development* (pp. 43–56). Jossey-Bass.

Higgins, L. (2012). *Community music: In theory and in practice.* Oxford University Press.

Hjørnevik, K., & Waage, L. (2019). The prison as a therapeutic music scene: Exploring musical identities in music therapy and everyday life in a prison setting. *Punishment & Society, 21*(4), 454–472.

Hochschild, A. R. (1983). *The managed heart: Commercialisation of human feeling.* University of California Press.

Holstein, J. A., & Gubrium, J. F. (2007). Constructionist perspectives on the life course. *Sociology Compass, 1*(1), 335–352.

Hooper, S., & Procter, S. (2013). Less comfortably numb, more meaningfully occupied. In E. Ruud, M. Skanland, & G. Trondalen (Eds.), *Musical life stories: Narratives on health musicking* (pp. 221–240). Norwegian Academy of Music.

Huynh, T., Alderson, M., & Thompson, M. (2008). Emotional labour underlying caring: An evolutionary concept analysis. *Journal of Advanced Nursing, 64*(2), 195–208.

Koen, B. (Ed.). (2012). *The Oxford handbook of medical ethnomusicology.* Oxford University Press.

Korczynski, M., Pickering, M., & Robertson, E. (2013). *Rhythms of labour: Music at work in Britain.* Cambridge University Press.

Kravits, K., McAllister-Black, R., Grant, M., & Kirk, C. (2010). Self-care strategies for nurses: A psycho-educational intervention for stress reduction and the prevention of burnout. *Applied Nursing Research, 23*(3), 130–138.

Kumm, B. E. (2013). Finding healing through songwriting: A song for Nicolette. *International Journal of Community Music, 6*(2), 205–217.

Lamont, A., Murray, M., Hale, R., & Wright-Bevans, K. (2018). Singing in later life: The anatomy of a community choir. *Psychology of Music, 46*(3), 424–439.

Langer, E. J. (2009). *Counterclockwise: Mindful health and the power of possibility.* Ballantine Books.

MacDonald, R. A. R. (2013). Music, health, and well-being: A review. *International Journal of Qualitative Studies on Health and Wellbeing, 8:* Article 20635. https://doi.org/10.3402/qhw.v8i0.20635

MacDonald, R., Hargreaves, D. J., & Miell, D. (Eds.). (2017). *Handbook of musical identities.* Oxford University Press.

McFerran, K. S., & Saarikallio, S. (2014). Depending on music to feel better: Being conscious of responsibility when appropriating the power of music. *The Arts in Psychotherapy, 41*(1), 89–97.

McKee, M., & Stuckler, D. (2012). The crisis of capitalism and the marketisation of health care: The implications for public health professionals. *Journal of Public Health Research*, *1*(3), 236–239.

Moss, H., Lynch, J., & O'Donoghue, J. (2018). Exploring the perceived health benefits of singing in a choir: An international cross-sectional mixed-methods study. *Perspectives in Public Health*, *138*(3), 160–168.

Nordberg, C. (2016) Outsourcing equality: Migrant care worker imaginary in Finnish media. *Nordic Journal of Working Life Studies*, *6*(3), 101–118.

Palmer, E., & Eveline, J. (2012). Sustaining low pay in aged care work. *Gender, Work and Organization*, *19*(3), 254–275.

Peller, L. E. (1946) Incentives to development and means of early education. *The Psychoanalytic Study of the Child*, *2*(1), 397–415.

Pilcher, J., Williams, J., & Pole, C. (2003). Rethinking adulthood: Families, transitions, and social change. *Sociological Research Online*, *8*(4), 181–185. https://doi.org/10.5153/sro.865

Pitman, A., Krysinska, K., & King, M. (2012). Suicide in young men. *The Lancet, 379*, 2383–2392.

Plumb, L., & Stickley, T. (2017). Singing to promote mental health and well-being. *Mental Health Practice*, *20*(8), 31–36.

Procter, S. (2011). Reparative musicing: Thinking on the usefulness of social capital theory within music therapy. *Nordic Journal of Music Therapy*, *20*(3), 242–262.

Ruud, E. (2008). Music in therapy: Increasing possibilities for action. *Music and Arts in Action, 1*(1), 46–60.

Skånland, M. S. (2013). Everyday music listening and affect regulation: The role of MP3 players. *International Journal of Qualitative Studies on Health and Well-being*, *8*(1): Article 20595. https://doi.org/10.3402/qhw.v8i0.20595

Sloboda, J. (2010). Music in everyday life: The role of emotions. In P. N. Juslin & J. Sloboda (Eds.), *Handbook of music and emotion: Theory, research, applications* (pp. 493–514). Oxford University Press.

Small, C. (1998). *Musicking: The meanings of performing and listening.* University Press of New England.

Theodosius, C. (2008). *Emotional labour in health care: The unmanaged heart of nursing.* Routledge.

Trevarthen, C. (2002). Origins of musical identity: Evidence from infancy for musical social awareness. In R. MacDonald, D. Hargreaves, & D. Miell (Eds.), *Musical identities* (pp. 21–38). Oxford University Press.

Tuastad, L., & Stige, B. (2018). Music as a way out: How musicking helped a collaborative rock band of ex-inmates. *British Journal of Music Therapy*, *32*(1), 27–37.

Williams, F. (2012). Converging variations in migrant care work in Europe. *Journal of European Social Policy*, *22*(4), 363–376.

Williamson, V., & Bonshor, M. (2019). Wellbeing in brass bands: The benefits and challenges of group music making. *Frontiers in Psychology*, *10*, 1176.

Wood S. (2020). Beyond Messiaen's birds: The post-verbal world of dementia. *Medical Humanities*, *46*, 73–83.

Zelic, K., Galic, I., Nedeljkovic, N., Jakovljevic, A., Milosevic, O., Djuric, M., & Cameriere, R. (2016). Accuracy of Cameriere's third molar maturity index in assessing legal adulthood on Serbian population. *Forensic Science International*, *259*, 127–132.

5
Musical care in older adulthood

A score for healthy ageing

Stuart Wood and Stephen Clift

Introduction

The dominant discourse connecting music and older people is one of 'healthy ageing', in which musical participation is recommended in the belief that it can help older people stay healthy and independent (APPG, 2107; Bowell and Bamford, 2018). To that end, a growing number of health and social initiatives are adopting music-based strategies, and policy-oriented discussions are highlighting the role of music for health in the wider context for promoting an 'arts, health and well-being' agenda. These include social prescribing (Bickerdike et al., 2016), promotion of the healthy or friendly environment (Kirklin and Richardson, 2003), professionalized medical and therapeutic interventions (Dileo, 1999), advances in care communication (Wood, 2017), national singing initiatives such as Choir in Every Care Home (Clift et al., 2017), and health practices such as Singing for Lung Health (Lewis, et al., 2016).

These initiatives pose the idea that forms of musical care might help address common health and social challenges. This chapter, written by a music therapist (Stuart Wood) and a health promotion specialist interested in music and health (Stephen Clift), explores, from a combined perspective, how music can be employed as a strategy of health and social care in older adulthood with individuals, groups, and communities.

Following an account of the current challenges in the United Kingdom associated with an ageing population and responses to it, the chapter goes on to discuss the idea of 'musical care' as part of the response to these challenges. We survey recent research on group singing as an intervention for older people living with long-term health complications, with particular reference to chronic obstructive pulmonary disease (COPD). The chapter then discusses musical care in the context of nursing and music therapy interventions, particularly with reference to dementia. In this section, a number of emergent aspects of such care are addressed: 'post-verbal' communication; music-therapeutic caregiving; musical care in care environments. The final section includes two case examples of our own work. The first symptom-specific intervention concerns singing and respiratory illness, describing the experience of a married couple, one of whom lives with COPD, participating in a singing-for-breathing

Stuart Wood and Stephen Clift, *Musical care in older adulthood* In: *Collaborative Insights.* Edited by: Neta Spiro and Katie Rose M. Sanfilippo, Oxford University Press. © Oxford University Press 2022. DOI: 10.1093/oso/9780197535011.003.0006 initiative (SC). The second tells the experiences of a woman in residential care who was working with the author, a music therapist (SW). Finally, the concluding sections propose future directions for research and suggest that imagination, collaboration, and care amongst musical practitioners may ensure that older adulthood remains a time of flourishing.

The UK ageing population and responses to the challenge

The global population (United Nations, 2019) is ageing, and this is presenting considerable challenges in the context of the United Kingdom for individuals, families, the National Health Service, local authorities, and the private health and social care sectors. Average life expectancy has climbed inexorably in the post–World War II period. In 1951, life expectancy at birth in the United Kingdom was 66.4 years for males and 71.5 years for females. In contrast, in 2014–2016, a newborn baby boy could expect to live 79.2 years and a baby girl 82.9 years. More importantly, given the focus of this chapter, a man aged 65 in 2014–2016 could expect to live on average a further 18.5 years, and a woman would have 20.9 years remaining (ONS, 2017).

With longer life spans has come an increasing burden of ill health, associated with lifestyle factors and genetic causes. These include coronary disease, lung disease, diabetes, dementias, and obesity. Problems associated with wear and tear on the body and its systems are also increasingly prevalent, including arthritis, hearing loss, and sight problems. Examples include the following:

- 7.8% of adults over the age of 75 experience lung disease, including COPD, chronic bronchitis, and emphysema (BLF, 2016).
- 23.8% of adults aged 75 years and over are affected by diabetes (PHE, 2016).
- 422,000 people aged 65 and over in England have a recorded dementia diagnosis affecting 1 person in 6 over 80 and 1 in 3 over 95 (Age UK, 2018).

A further significant consideration is that problems of chronic disease are socially distributed and social inequalities in health increase with age. Socio-economic inequalities in ill health and disability typically take the form of 'social gradients' with higher socio-economic groups having better health and fewer disabilities than lower socio-economic groups (Marmot, 2010). Furthermore, an important distinction should be drawn between life expectancy and healthy life expectancy, with this gap increasing as communities become more economically disadvantaged (Marmot, 2010).

Faced with these challenges, health services in the United Kingdom are undergoing a fundamental shift towards placing greater emphasis on prevention and health promotion—to do more to help people lead healthier lives, and so remain free from serious illness and able to live independently for longer. This emphasis builds upon a tradition of 'up-stream' thinking that goes back several decades and was enshrined on an international level by the World Health Organization initially in the Ottawa Charter (WHO, 1986).

There is too an increased awareness of non-medical/non-pharmacological ways of helping people to manage long-term conditions more effectively, so that even when health problems develop, there are still advantages to maintaining a 'healthy lifestyle' as far as is possible, through exercise, good diet, not smoking, moderate drinking, and attention to rest and sleep. This awareness is reflected in the growth of interest in 'social prescribing', which seeks to signpost patients to opportunities for increasing physical, social, and creative engagement for improved health and well-being (Crone et al., 2018; Polley et al., 2017).

Primary and secondary health promotion provides a context for understanding the growth of interest in the United Kingdom since 2000 in the power of the arts and creative activity in promoting health in both communities and health care settings. Such initiatives complement the already well-established creative arts therapies, and the provision, within the context of health and social care services, of therapeutic interventions through the arts, movement, drama, and music. Arts for health and well-being initiatives, however, stand in contrast to specifically focused creative arts therapeutic interventions, as they may be led by non-therapeutically trained arts practitioners or musicians. Both approaches have in common the assumption that engaging in quality creative, artistic, or musical activity, individually or with other people, is inherently beneficial for a sense of well-being and may have specific benefits for health.

The degree to which the field of 'arts, health and well-being' has established itself in the United Kingdom is indicated by the growth of reports, the appearance of specialist journals, the publication of textbooks, the creation of national awards, and the development of professional and research networks (Clift et al., 2009; Clift and Camic, 2015; Fancourt, 2017; Stickley, et al., 2016). A recent major landmark has been the publication of *Creative Health*, by the All Party Parliamentary Group for Arts, Health and Wellbeing (APPG, 2017). This report provides a life course perspective on arts and health and gives a comprehensive overview of arts for health interventions across the United Kingdom, including for older people.

Applications of musical care

Our approach to the notion of musical care reflects our interdisciplinary stance, and our shared belief that music touches upon aspects of care at micro (within individuals), meso (amongst groups and institutions), and macro (society and culture at large) levels. Indeed, we observe in our research, practice, and teaching that the micro detail of musical interaction has implications at the most broad macro-cultural level, and that issues of global culture and aesthetics impact upon how individuals experience music even in their most solitary moments (Pavlicevic et al, 2015). Musical care experiences inevitably generate both individual functional change and social or cultural activity (Wood and Crow, 2018), and the inherent character of music serves to bring people together both within themselves, and amongst one another, simultaneously. Musical care involves the use of music specifically as an intervention within care settings, as well as the musical awareness involved in everyday nonverbal communication, the attention paid to the acoustic of care environments, and the care we take as practitioners and researchers in our musical work.

In the following sections we explore interrelated aspects of musical care in working with older people: firstly, we focus on the value for older people of coming together to sing, and secondly, we look at musical care and music therapy practices in health and social care settings.

Singing, well-being, and health

Since 2000 there has been a tremendous growth of interest in the value of singing across the United Kingdom. In part this can be attributed to the 'Gareth Malone' effect—the influence of the BBC series of programmes called 'The Choir' in which Gareth Malone has created choirs in a wide variety of settings and with people from all walks of life, with little or no background in music or singing (The Workplace Choir, 2017).

Increasingly, too, it is recognized that giving older people the opportunity to come together to sing functions as a form of caring that can have important positive benefits for their sense of personal and social well-being and can even help to ameliorate health problems. This benefit is reflected in the growth of projects promoting singing in communities for older people with specific health conditions, including

- Singing for the Brain, for people with dementias and their carers, supported by the Alzheimer's Society https://www.alzheimers.org.uk/info/20172/your_support_services/765/singing_for_the_brain
- Singing for Lung Health, for people with COPD and other lung conditions, supported by the British Lung Foundation https://www.blf.org.uk/support-for-you/singing-for-lung-health
- Sing to Beat Parkinson's, for people affected by Parkinson's, devised and promoted by the Canterbury Cantata Trust https://canterburycantatatrust.org.uk/our-choirs/sing-to-beat-parkinson-s
- Sing with Us Choirs, for people affected by cancer, organized and delivered by the cancer charity Tenovus http://www.tenovuscancercare.org.uk/singwithus

Currently, there are also considerable efforts being made by Live Music Now, to promote the value of group singing in all care settings across the United Kingdom through 'A Choir in Every Care Home': https://achoirineverycarehome.wordpress.com/.

How does 'caring' through singing for older people with long-term progressive conditions work? It has to be said, firstly, that no amount of singing is going to cure people of conditions like dementia, Parkinson's, COPD, or cancer, although it may in some cases help to ameliorate symptoms or give people a greater sense of control over their condition. But what it can certainly do is help to promote a greater sense of personal and social well-being and give a sense of purpose and achievement that can add to quality of life (see, for example, Clements-Cortes, 2013; Johnson et al., 2013). Part of the reason for this result can be understood by contrasting such musical care with common aspects of health or medical care for these conditions, in which the focus is generally on the individual and the declining function of specific bodily systems (whether in relation to cognition, lung function, strength and coordination, or speech), and prescribing pharmacological or surgical interventions. Engaging people with a common health problem in singing, in contrast, involves bringing people together socially, and supporting a positive, enjoyable engagement with music, with a focus on what people can do, and with practice can do increasingly well.

These ideas are explored in greater detail by focusing on the value of singing for people with respiratory illness. Recent research on this topic is briefly reviewed here and an illustrative case study is given in a later section of the chapter of one couple's experiences of engaging in a singing project for people affected by COPD in East Kent (Morrison, et al., 2013).

Singing and respiratory illness

COPD is a preventable disease characterized by persistent respiratory symptoms and airflow limitation (GOLD, 2017; RCP, 2016). The most common symptoms include breathlessness and cough with sputum. The major causes are smoking, air pollution, and other environmental exposures. COPD is progressive and incurable, but it can be managed. Both drug therapy and pulmonary rehabilitation can improve exercise capacity and psychological well-being, and reduce breathlessness (NICE, 2016). The benefits gained from structured exercise-based rehabilitation tend to fade, however, unless people maintain activity and social engagement (BTS, 2013), and one activity that may be helpful for people with COPD as part of a managed programme of care is group singing.

Four small trials on singing and COPD have found mixed and generally non-significant results in objective physical measures (e.g., lung volumes, breath hold times, walk test, exercise capacity) following singing programmes (Bonilha et al., 2009; Goodridge et al., 2013; Lord et al., 2010, 2012). However, these studies were based on small samples, and were likely to be underpowered for detecting real changes. Morrison et al. (2013), in contrast, found significant improvements in respiratory measures, in a non-randomized, observational study, although this finding was not confirmed by a further non-randomized study that attempted to replicate the Morrison et al. study (Skingley, et al., 2018). A systematic review (Lewis, et al., 2016), and the more recent Cochrane review (McNamara et al., 2017), have both concluded that the existing evidence of the effectiveness of singing in relation to lung function in COPD patients is limited, although the qualitative evidence based on participant feedback is very encouraging.

Some studies have gathered written comments from participants, which capture broader dimensions of well-being than can be assessed through physiological measures and standardized questionnaires alone. Goodridge et al. (2013), in a study of singing as an adjunct to pulmonary rehabilitation, reported feedback from the 14 members of a therapeutic singing group and highlighted feelings of pleasure, being uplifted, relaxation, learning to manage breathing and social benefits. A larger study by Skingley et al. (2014) gathered written comments from participants taking part in a singing for breathing programme. The feedback indicated perceived improvements in quality of life, control of breathing problems, and social well-being. Lord et al. (2010, 2012) undertook interviews with participants who reported improvements in breathing, general well-being, posture, social support, and achievement. In a further study (BLF, 2017) interview and focus group data confirmed that participants experienced physical, social, and psychological benefits from participating in singing groups.

McNaughton et al. (2016, 2017) also conducted interviews and a focus group discussion with participants with COPD engaging in singing. Themes emerging from the qualitative data included improvements to breathing and emphasized the importance of the social aspects of the singing group, even though few of the quantitative measures showed changes. A similar pattern of findings also emerged from a recent larger-scale non-controlled study of group singing in South London, a study that again found no changes in respiratory function, but very clear and positive reported benefits for control of breathlessness and social and psychological well-being (Clift, et al., 2017a; Skingley et al., 2018).

The existing body of evidence appears to support the potential value of regular singing for people with COPD, but points to the clear need for further larger-scale controlled trials. Future studies need to employ techniques of assessment better attuned to measuring changes that occur in the patterns and efficiency of breath control and use of the lungs (in particular a shift from upper thoracic, shallow breathing to deeper breathing with long out-breaths supported by the diaphragm), rather than relatively crude assessments of overall lung capacity. They also need to incorporate the equally important psychological and social effects of group singing in older adulthood.

Musical care approaches in dementia

This section considers the role that musical care can play in health care and social care environments, whether provided by professional musicians, music therapists, or health and social care staff. Of particular relevance in this context is the work of Malloch and Trevarthen (2009) on the inherent 'musicality' of everyday interaction, and the role 'communicative musicality' plays in parent-child interaction in the earliest 'preverbal' years of life (as discussed in more detail in the Musical care in infancy chapter). Communicative musicality can be also applied in the examination of the role of music in later life, especially where older people may find verbal communication difficult. Indeed, Wood (2017, 2020) has applied these notions of the musicality of everyday interaction in the context of music therapy with older people as a form of 'post-verbal' communication.

Though core works in the field of communicative musicality acknowledge the value of musical terminology in describing preverbal interactions, scant work has been done to advance what has been termed 'post-verbal' interactions (Wood, 2020), such as the interactions that occur with people living in later stages of dementia. Existing literature on nursing and care in dementia care consistently identifies this aspect of practice as highly sensitive and often leading to anxiety or alienation both on the part of the carer and the cared for (Eggenberger et al., 2013).

One significant factor in these reactions is the trauma inherent in the loss of verbal communication as a mode of creating meaning. Smaller pockets of nursing research identify nonverbal communication (Caris-Verhallen et al. 1999) to be a helpful means of alleviating that trauma. Dementia care communication is rooted in musical aspects such as rhythmic matching in vocal sound effects, pitch attunement in vocalization, voiced signals of empathy and activity, and the use of significant songs or musical fragments as orientating devices (Miell et al., 2005). Research indicates the potential impact of music therapy on language function in dementia care (Brotons and Kroger, 2000).

Dementia care relies on expressive vocal components to build relationships and carry meaning, often taking precedence over the semantic content of words. For example, dementia care communication is influenced significantly by the impact of emotional tone. Willams and Herman (2011) demonstrate that emotional tone is an influencing factor in creating resistance to care in dementia care settings. Ward et al. (2008) also make a strong case that communication is a contested area of dementia care. The authors claim that communication is at the heart of person-centred dementia care, and yet people with dementia can be excluded from person-centred care through inappropriate communication methods. They also suggest that medical education and care training should reflect better approaches to dementia care communication. This claim is also at the core of Kitwood's interpersonal approach to dementia care (Kitwood, 1993). It may be that future approaches to dementia care communication will make use of musical terminology more fully, and indeed that music therapy may become a more active partner in addressing the traumas of language loss.

A significant allied field in relation to the musicality of dementia care communication is the literature on 'Music-Therapeutic Care-Giving'. Brown et al., (2001) argue for the necessity of music-making as part of clinical care. This signposts a body of literature on the impact of caregivers' singing, also briefly discussed in the previous chapter on Musical care in adulthood, in relation to a range of everyday events in dementia care, including the use of background music in social situations (Götell et al., 2002), use of voice to help with person transfer moments (Götell et al., 2012), singing during morning care routines (Hammar et al., 2011), and the role of music in transcending the limits of institutionalization (Allison, 2011). By including musical activities such as singing or by paying close attention to ambient sounds and silences during personal care or mealtimes, care workers and nurses may counteract some of the task focus that is inherent in modern care culture. Music challenges institutionalization not only for the older person but also for the health professional and the workplace. This challenge creates an opportunity to address the role of music in older peoples' care not only as a specialist recreational activity delivered by appointed 'experts' but also as a necessary dimension of everyday interaction.

Music-making has a positive impact upon care environments (Pavlicevic et al., 2015; Ragneskog et al., 1996). Artistic activity changes how older people are viewed within those environments, often enhancing their active ability to make change and contribute. As the following case study will illustrate, this enhancement can extend beyond the care environment into the life of the local community (Wood, 2016). It has been shown that music-making has an impact on the attitudes of care staff towards people living with dementia (Sung et al., 2011). Musical care may indeed be a currency that older people contribute to society, and not only receive.

Case examples of musical care in older adulthood

Alongside the ecological view of arts in health previously set out, in some instances music is adopted in a more causative strategy, towards symptom-specific change in clinical terms. For example, this is well illustrated by music therapy's application in behaviour and emotional regulation within dementia care. Research indicates that music therapy can be effective in the management of behavioural symptoms of dementia (Chang et al., 2015; Khan and Curtice, 2011; Ueda et al., 2013), and in the alleviation of apathy amongst people living with dementia (Holmes et al, 2006). Music therapy evidence shows the reduction of agitation and depression (Raglio et al., 2015; Ray and Mittelman, 2017; Ridder, 2013) amongst older people with dementia.

The aim of this book is to explore ways in which different methods and perspectives can be complementary in a holistic approach to musical care across the life course. In this penultimate section, therefore, we offer two case studies to illustrate concretely the benefits older people gain from engagement with music. In the first example, we describe experiences of a married couple, in their late 60s, in which the husband is living with COPD, who together join a singing for breathing project and discover the benefits that singing can bring physically, psychologically, and socially. The second example describes the journey of a care home resident from singing in a choir to composing her own musical works in music therapy with the author, for eventual public performance.

A case study of the benefits of singing for people with COPD

As previously outlined, Skingley et al. (2014, 2018) have reported two studies of singing and COPD, which have gathered qualitative feedback from participants. Sadly, in both studies, some participants have subsequently passed away as a result of exacerbations or complications associated with their lung disease. This loss highlights the point made earlier, that though singing may bring benefits in helping older people better manage their lung condition, and even ameliorate some symptoms, ageing and the underlying damage are progressive and inexorable, and no amount of singing will reverse the disease process. Nevertheless, the evidence from the experience of people participating in the groups is that singing can help with managing symptoms in daily life, improve quality of life, and widen a person's circle of social support and friendship.

All of these issues are reflected clearly in the following case study of Harry and Pamela. Harry was a keen supporter of his singing group in East Kent. He and his wife, Pamela, were actively involved in keeping the group going following the end of the research phase. Harry participated until his death, and Pamela continued to be part of the ongoing group to support friends. Here Harry and Pamela talk about the benefits that Harry experienced from joining a singing group.

Harry, described the origins of his COPD, and his diagnosis:

I've got COPD and it developed through smoking from when I was 13 for 50 years. Plus, I worked in the building trade as a plasterer, so I was exposed to a lot of dust, one way or another, most of my working life. So that doesn't help. Then suddenly ... yes, suddenly, COPD got a hold of me. I just thought I was smoking too much, but that wasn't the case. My lungs were damaged beyond repair. I stopped smoking, but it didn't make any difference. So since then, I've just been [doing] anything I can to improve my lot, to be honest.

I went for tests, usual tests of blowing and the usual business. I've not had bad treatment, I just went through all the necessary checks, and then my doctor said er, I went to get the results, and he said: 'You've got COPD, and it will kill you, or something related to it.' So that was it. And it is doing, slowly, I go worse each year. But er, you just live with it a day at a time. I'm not worried at all. I enjoy my life, I can tell you, a lot more than a lot of other people.

Pamela describes joining a singing group together, and the benefits she has seen in Harry:

We heard about the group and felt that it would be beneficial to come to that group if it was going to help his breathing and his well-being all together, as well as mixing socially with other people of like illness. He looks forward to coming. Whereas some things that we do, perhaps, it's a little bit of 'Oh, do we need to?' Instead of that, he doesn't. He looks forward to coming, erm, and he really does say, and I'm not just saying this to you [the interviewer], he really does say: 'You know, I feel a lot better for going, I really do, my breathing's better.' And then of course, socially, he's made so many friends. That's it! All in all, it's a good thing to do, and we do it together.

Harry confirms the benefits of singing, both in the sessions, and outside them in daily life:

It does definitely help me to clear my chest. Even when I come in here, sometimes, especially when the weather has been a bit cold, my chest's a bit tight, but once we've done some warming up exercises, my chest clears. So then I started taking that with me, outside of singing, and it helps me all through my life really, when I walk up stairs, or walking around shopping centres, anything like that, I still use the exercises I've learned here.

Pamela further elaborates on the impacts of COPD on Harry, and on the benefits of maintaining activity and engagement:

It's very demoralizing not being able to do what you could do a few years ago, and everything is an effort, you know. You can't walk like you used to, and it's so restricting, and so I think, yes, any of these things that can avoid hospitalization, and more and more drug treatment, I think can only be good.

These comments come from a film about the East Kent project, which can be viewed here: https://www.youtube.com/watch?v=c0UK2X3i-FU. The film contains an account of the project and how it was evaluated, together with testimonials from a number of participants.

'Five Seasons'

Caryl (it was Caryl's express wish that her real name be used in any writing about her experiences) was a mature woman in her 60s who was living with cerebral palsy in a care home in southern England. Although Caryl's mind and insight were undiminished, her body was severely limited by the effects of her condition. Spending her days in an adapted wheelchair, Caryl was able to use only her right foot, usually with it resting on a control switch, but sometimes with her leg extended for short periods. She spent six months in individual music therapy. After that time, a new phase of work began in which she wrote a choral song cycle that was performed in a local church by a choir.

Caryl referred herself to individual music therapy. She was not interested in combating symptoms of a specific diagnosis, but rather in answering a personal question brought on by the advance of years: 'What can I still do?' My initial question for Caryl was also to find out what she could do: to understand her physical strength, flexibility, control, and range. It was important for me also to understand how Caryl used these abilities; I aimed to meet her style of musicality, in order to be fully open to what she would bring.

In her verbal feedback, Caryl gave some clues about what was valuable to her personally:

> I've always wanted to play the piano ... I never thought I would play it. I'm losing the feeling in my foot so I can't do anything—but it doesn't matter with this. I go by hearing my music.

Gradually a new sense of musical purpose emerged: to achieve a lifelong ambition, to defy the effects of her disease in the context of ageing, and to enhance her pleasure in life. Assisted by foam supports supplied by her physiotherapist, Caryl used her foot to play not only the piano, but also the drum, cymbal, and numerous other percussion instruments. Her exploration had a multifaceted impact while being guided by an artistic motivation.

When Caryl said that she had started to write poems that she wanted to be set to music, she entered a new phase of work. She now spent her evenings in thinking of poems and memorizing them. During her sessions, she recited the poems and I transcribed them for her as song lyrics. We then improvised melodies to go with the poems. This compositional approach was in part a pragmatic response to Caryl's increasing difficulty in forming flowing speech, which had been exacerbated by the ongoing effects of her cerebral palsy. By transferring the prosodic elements of speech into musical melody and phrasing, Caryl was able to harness the post-verbal affordances of music and maintain her expressiveness.

Caryl's lyrics dealt with reminiscence, nostalgia, life lessons, and a love of nature. As this process continued, Caryl's confidence and skills grew, to the extent that musical activity was no longer confined to the workroom, nor to her time with me. She sang solos in the care home's cabaret shows, did musical voice exercises every morning with her carer, and took more interest in musical history through her recreational listening. She was living more fully as a musical person throughout her life. From our initial questions, a concrete goal had manifested: to complete a set of songs, arrange them for a choir, and then have a performance. Caryl's first song cycle, 'Five Seasons', was eventually performed in her local church by a community choir to an audience of church members, friends, staff, and family.

The lyrics from one song reflect Caryl's blend of reminiscence and philosophy:

> I remember autumn
> Many years ago

Crunching through the leaves along the path
Clouds would break above me
Showing me the sun
Then the rains would come—and I would laugh!
The nights are getting longer
The days are getting colder
But we just wrap up warmer . . .

Leaves grow
Leaves turn
Leaves fall
. . . and grow again

It seems misrepresentative of older people for them to be identified as only the recipient of musical care and not in many cases the provider of it. In Caryl's experience music was a way of exploring long-held ambitions, and of maintaining a sense of self that had been built through strenuous effort over adulthood. Caryl's sense of self involved a significant ethic of contribution, and music became a means of fulfilling that. She appreciated being able to entertain, bring pleasure, and perhaps prompt valuable reflection in others, through her singing and her writing. It is perhaps implicit in such experiences that music is a mode in which giving is rarely one-directional, creating instead a dynamic in which giving truly is receiving—and vice versa.

Case studies of the kind presented in this section provide a valuable complement to research evidence that focuses on group outcomes from musical programmes. Where these outcomes are based on quantitative assessments it is very easy to lose sight of the processes and individuals involved—and it is these essential qualitative aspects of the work that come to the fore when we hear the direct testimony that comes from people on their experience of engaging with music and the benefits they gain.

Future directions

Our approach to the notion of musical care reflects our interdisciplinary stance, and our shared belief that music touches upon aspects of care at micro, meso, and macro levels. For future research it is essential that qualitative experiences are prioritized through hearing the direct testimony that comes from people on their experience of engaging with music and the benefits they gain. Though no amount of musical care is going to cure people of conditions like dementia, Parkinson's, COPD, or cancer, in some cases it can help to ameliorate symptoms, or give people a greater sense of control over their condition. What it can certainly do is help to promote a greater sense of personal and social well-being, and give a sense of purpose and achievement that can add to quality of life. However, as is common across many parts of musical care, there is still scope for outcomes based on systematic investigations of associations between music engagement for particular purposes and specific outcomes (like lung function in COPD). In addition, future approaches to communication in dementia care could helpfully make use of musical terminology more fully, helping to address the traumas of language loss.

More broadly, there can often be a large drop in participation in arts activities after discharge from hospital, mainly because of physical access, loss of confidence, and loss of motivation. Helpful in this context is the notion of 'aesthetic health'. Moss and O'Neill develop their concept of aesthetics in medicine, proposing a notion of aesthetic deprivation (2014). This deprivation includes ideas related to artistic interests and passions amongst older people; the impact of loss of aesthetic and leisure interests; low expectation of artistic standards in hospital; the aesthetic components of hospital stays; how the benefits of arts in hospital are considered and communicated; aims and outcomes for arts interventions in hospitals. Future work should explore how involvement in cultural, artistic, or 'aesthetic' experiences could be useful in health assessment.

Conclusions

The dominant discourse connecting music and older people is one of 'healthy ageing', in which musical participation is recruited in the belief that it can help older people stay healthy and independent. In addition, it is clear that as older people move from the third to the fourth ages of life (Gilleard & Higgs, 2014), they progress from an era of possible personal fulfilment to a period of dependency requiring social and nursing care. In this shift, music can also help to maintain quality of life if used with imagination and collaboration. The growing number of social and political approaches that adopt music-based strategies within them demonstrate the potential for interdisciplinary and international collaboration. These emerging strategies pose the challenge of evidencing how musical care might help address common health and social problems. Imaginative and collaborative approaches to musical care in older adulthood, including creative practices in nursing, care, and therapy, attention to the social environment of care, and continued careful practice amongst musical practitioners, may ensure that older adulthood remains a time of flourishing.

References

Age UK (2018). *Later life in the United Kingdom*. https://www.ageuk.org.uk/globalassets/age-uk/documents/reports-and-publications/later_life_uk_factsheet.pdf

Allison, T. (2011) Transcending the limitations of institutionalization through music: Ethnomusicology in a Nursing Home. PhD Diss. University of Illinois.

APPG (2017). *Creative health: The arts for health and wellbeing*. All Party Parliamentary Group for Arts, Health and Wellbeing. http://www.artshealthandwellbeing.org.uk/appg-inquiry/Publications/Creative_Health_Inquiry_Report_2017.pdf

Bickerdike, L., Booth, A., Wilson, P., Farley, K., & Wright, K. (2016). Social prescribing: less rhetoric and more reality: A systematic review of the evidence. *BMJ Open 7*: e013384. doi:10.1136/bmjopen-2016-013384.

BLF (2016). *The battle for breath*. British Lung Foundation. https://cdn.shopify.com/s/files/1/0221/4446/files/The_Battle_for_Breath_report_48b7e0ee-dc5b-43a0-a25c-2593bf9516f4.pdf?7045701451358472254

BLF (2017). *BLF Singing Project report*. London: British Lung Foundation.

Bonilha, A. G., Onofre, F., Vieira, L. M., Prado, M. Y. A., & Martinez, J. A. B. (2009). Effects of singing classes on pulmonary function and quality of life of COPD patients. *International Journal of COPD, 4*(1), 1–8.

Bowell, S., & Bamford, S. M. (2018). *What would life be—Without a song and a dance, what are we?* International Longevity Centre.

Brotons, M., & Koger, S. M. (2000). The impact of music therapy on language functioning in dementia. *Journal of Music Therapy. 37*(3), 183–195.

Brown, S., Götell, E., & Ekman, S. (2001). 'Music-therapeutic caregiving': The necessity of active music-making in clinical care. *Arts in Psychotherapy, 28*(2), 125–135.

Bolton C. E., Bevan-Smith E. F., Blakey J. D., Crowe P., Elkin S. L., Garrod R., Greening N. J., Heslop K., Hull J. H., Man W. D., & Morgan M. D. (2013). British Thoracic Society guideline on pulmonary rehabilitation in adults: accredited by NICE. *Thorax, 68*(2), ii1–ii30.

Caris-Verhallen, W. M. C. M., Kerkstra, A., & Bensing, J. M. (1999). Non-verbal behaviour in nurse–elderly patient communication. *Journal of Advanced Nursing, 29,* 4,808–818.

Chang, Y. S., Chu, H., Yang, C. Y., et al. (2015). The efficacy of music therapy for people with dementia: A meta-analysis of randomised controlled trials. *Journal of Clinical Nursing, 24,* 3425–3440.

Clements-Cortes, A. A. (2013). Buddy's Glee Club: Singing for life. *Adaptation & Aging, 37*(4), 273–290.

Clift, S., Camic, P., Chapman, B., Clayton, G., Daykin, N., Eades, G., Parkinson, C., Secker, J., Stickley, T., & White, M. (2009). The state of arts and health in England. *Arts and Health: An International Journal for Research, Policy and Practice, 1*(1), 6–35.

Clift, S., and Camic, P. (Eds). (2015). *Oxford textbook for creative arts, health and wellbeing.* Oxford University Press.

Clift, S., Gilbert, R., & Vella-Burrows, T. (2017a). Health and well-being benefits of singing for older people. In N. Sutherland, N. Lewandowski, and B. Bendrups (Eds.), *Music, health and wellbeing: Exploring music for health equity and social justice* (pp. 97–120). Springer.

Clift, S., Skingley, A., Page, S., et al. (2017b). *Singing for better breathing: Findings from the Lambeth and Southwark singing and COPD Project.* Canterbury Christ Church University.

Crone, D., Sumner, R. C., Baker, C. M., Loughren, E. A., Hughes, S., & James, D. V. (2018). 'Artlift' arts-on-referral intervention in UK primary care: Updated findings from an ongoing observational study. *European Journal of Public Health, 28*(3), 404–409.

Dileo, C. (1999). *Music therapy and medicine: Theoretical and clinical applications.* American Music Therapy Association.

Eggenberger, E., Heimerl, K., & Bennett, M. (2013). Communication skills training in dementia care: A systematic review of effectiveness, training content, and didactic methods in different care settings. *International Psychogeriatrics 25*(3), 345–358.

Fancourt. D. (2017). *Arts and health: Designing and evaluating interventions.* Oxford University Press.

Gilleard, C., & Higgs, P. (2014). Third and fourth ages. In W. C. Cockerham, R. Dingwall, & S. Quah (Eds.), *The Wiley Blackwell encyclopedia of health, illness, behavior, and society.* Wiley.

GOLD (2017). *Pocket guide to COPD diagnosis, management and prevention.* Global Initiative for Chronic Obstructive Lung Disease

Goodridge D., Nicol, J., Horvey, K., & Butcher, S. (2013). Therapeutic singing as an adjunct for pulmonary rehabilitation participants with COPD: Outcomes of a feasibility study. *Music and Medicine, 5*(3), 169–176.

Götell, E., Brown, S., & Ekman, S. (2002). Caregiver singing and background music in dementia care. *Western Journal of Nursing Research, 24*, 195–216.

Götell, E., Thunborg, C., Söderlund, A., & Heideken Wågert, P. (2012). Can caregiver singing improve person transfer situations in dementia care? *Music and Medicine, 4*(4), 237–244.

Hammar, L. M., Emami, A., Götell, E., & Engström, G. (2011). The impact of caregivers' singing on expressions of emotion and resistance during morning care situations in persons with dementia: An intervention in dementia care. *Journal of Clinical Nursing, 20*(7–8), 969–978.

Holmes, C., Knights, A., Dean, C., Hodkinson, S., & Hopkins, V. (2006). Keep music live: Music and the alleviation of apathy in dementia subjects. *International Psychogeriatrics, 18*(4), 623–630.

Johnson, J., Louhivuori, J., Stewart, A., Tolvanen, A., Ross, L., & Era, P. (2013). Quality of life (QOL) of older adult community choral singers in Finland. *International Psychogeriatrics, 25*(7), 1055–1064.

Khan, F., & Curtice, M. (2011). Non-pharmocological management of behavioural symptoms of dementia. *British Journal of Community Nursing, 16*(9), 441–449.

Kitwood, T. (1993). Towards a theory of dementia care: The interpersonal process. *Ageing and Society, 13*(1), 51–67.

Kirklin, D., & Richardson, R. (2003). *The healing environment: Without and within.* Royal College of Physicians.

Lewis, A., Cave, P., Stern, M., Welch, L., Taylor, K., Russell, J., Doyle, A. M., Russell, A. M., McKee, H., Clift, S., & Bott, J. (2016). Singing for Lung Health—A systematic review of the literature and consensus statement. *npj Primary Care Respiratory Medicine, 26*, 1–8. https://doi.org/10.1038/npjpcrm.2016.80

Lord, V. M., Cave, P., Hume, V., Flude, E. J., Evans, A., Kelly, J. L., Polkey, M. I., & Hopkinson, N. S. (2010). Singing teaching as a therapy for chronic respiratory disease—Randomised controlled trial and qualitative evaluation. *BMC Pulmonary Medicine, 10*, 41. https://doi.org/10.1186/1471-2466-10-41

Lord, V. M., Hume, V. J., Kelly, J. L., Cave, P., Silver, J., Waldman, M., White C., Smith C., Tanner R., Sanchez M., & Man W. D. (2012). Singing classes for chronic obstructive pulmonary disease: A randomized controlled trial. *BMC Pulmonary Medicine, 12*, 69. https://doi.org/10.1186/1471-2466-12-69

Malloch, S., & Trevarthen, C. (Eds.). (2009). *Communicative musicality: Exploring the casis of human companionship.* Oxford University Press.

Marmot, M. (2010). *Fair society, healthy lives.* Institute of Health Equity.

McNamara, R. J., Epsley, C., Coren, E., & McKeough, Z. J. (2017). Singing for adults with obstructive pulmonary disease (COPD). *Cochrane Database of Systematic Reviews.* http://doi.org/10.1002/14651858.CD012296.pub2.

McNaughton, A., Aldington, S., Williams, G., & Levack, W. M. (2016). Sing Your Lungs Out: A qualitative study of a community singing group for people with chronic obstructive pulmonary disease (COPD). *BMJ Open, 6*, 1–7. doi:10.1136/bmjopen-2016-012521.

McNaughton, A., Weatherall, M., Williams, M., McNaughton, H., Aldington, S., Williams, G., & Beasley, R. (2017). Sing Your Lungs Out: A community singing group for chronic obstructive pulmonary disease: A 1-year pilot study. *BMJ Open, 7*, 1–8. doi:10.1136/bmjopen-2016-014151.

Miell, D., MacDonald R., & Hargeaves, D. (2005). *Musical communication.* Oxford University Press.

Morrison, I., Clift, S., Page, S., Salisbury, I., Shipton, M., Skingley, A., Burrows, T.V., Coulton S., & Treadwell, P. (2013). A UK feasibility study on the value of singing for people with chronic obstructive pulmonary disease (COPD). *UNESCO Observatory Multi-Disciplinary Journal in the Arts, 3*(3),1–19.

Moss, H., & O'Neill, D. (2014). Aesthetic deprivation in clinical settings. *Lancet, 383,* 1032–1033.

NICE (2016). *Chronic obstructive pulmonary disease in adults: Quality statement* [updated February 2016]. National Institute for Health and Care Excellence.

ONS (2017). *National Life Tables, UK: 2014–2016.* Office of National Statistics.

Pavlicevic, M., Tsiris, G., Wood, S., Powell, H., Graham, J., Sanderson, R., Millman, R., & Gibson, J. (2015). The 'ripple effect': Towards researching improvisational music therapy in dementia care homes. *Dementia: The International Journal of Social Research and Practice, 14*(5), 659–679.

PHE (2016). *Diabetes prevalence model.* Public Health England.

Polley, M., Fleming, J., Anfilogoff, T., et al. (2017). *Making sense of social Prescribing.* University of Westminster.

Raglio, A., Bellandi, D., Baiardi, P., et al. (2015). Effect of active music therapy and individualized listening to music on dementia: A multicenter randomized controlled trial. *Journal of the American Geriatrics Society, 63*(8), 1534–1539.

Ragneskog, H., Bråne, G., Karlsson, I., & Kihlgren, M. (1996). Influence of dinner music on food intake and symptoms common in dementia. *Scandinavian Journal of Caring Sciences, 19*(1), 11–17.

Ray, K. D., & Mittelman, M. S. (2017). Music therapy: A nonpharmacological approach to the care of agitation and depressive symptoms for nursing home residents with dementia. *Dementia, 16*(7), 689–710.

RCP (2016). *COPD in England—Finding the measure of success* [National COPD Audit Programme]. Royal College of Physicians and Royal College of General Practitioners.

Ridder, H. (2013). Individual music therapy for agitation in dementia: An exploratory randomized controlled trial. *Aging and Mental Health, 17*(6), 667–678.

Skingley, A., Page, S., Clift, S., Morrison, I., Coulton, S., Treadwell, P., Vella-Burrows, T., Salisbury I., & Shipton, M. (2014). 'Singing for Breathing' groups for people with COPD: Participants' experiences. *Arts and Health: An International Journal for Research, Policy and Practice, 6*(2), 59–74.

Skingley, A., Clift, S., Hurley, S., Price, S., & Stephens, L. (2018). Community singing groups for people with chronic obstructive pulmonary disease: Participant perspectives. *Perspectives in Public Health, 138*(1), 66–75.

Stickley, T., Parr, H., Daykin, N., Stickley, T., Parr, H., Atkinson, S., Daykin, N., Clift, S., De Nora, T., Hacking, S., Camic, P. M., Joss, T., White, M., & Hogan, S. (2016). Arts, health and wellbeing: Reflections on a national seminar series and building a UK research network. *Arts and Health: An International Journal for Research, Policy and Practice, 9*(1), 14–25.

Sung, H.-C., Lee, W.-L., Chang, S.-M., & Smith, G.D. (2011). Exploring nursing staff's attitudes and use of music for older people with dementia in long-term care facilities. *Journal of Clinical Nursing, 20*(11–12), 1776–1783.

Ueda, T., Suzukamo, Y., Sato, M., & Izumi, S. (2013). Effects of music therapy on behavioral and psychological symptoms of dementia: A systematic review and meta-analysis. *Ageing Research Review, 12,* 628–641.

Ward, R., Vass, A., Aggarwal, N., Garfield, C., & Cybyk, B. (2008). A different story: Exploring patterns of communication in residential dementia care. *Ageing and Society, 28*(5), 629–651.

WHO (1986). *The Ottawa Charter.* http://www.who.int/healthpromotion/conferences/previous/ottawa/en/

Williams, K., & Herman, R. (2011). Linking resident behaviour to dementia care communication: Effects of emotional tone. *Behavior Therapy, 42*(1), 42–46.

Wood, S. (2016). *A matrix for community music therapy practice.* Barcelona Publishers.

Wood, S. (2017). 'Found performance': Towards a musical methodology for exploring the aesthetics of care. *Healthcare, 5*(3), 59. https://doi.org/10.3390/healthcare5030059.

Wood, S. (2020). Beyond Messiaen's birds: The post-verbal world of dementia. *BMJ Medical Humanities, 46,* 73–83.

Wood, S., & Crow, F. (2018) The music matrix: A qualitative participatory action research project to develop documentation for care home music therapy services. *British Journal of Music Therapy, 32*(2), 74–85.

The Work Place Choir (2017). The Gareth Malone Effect. http://www.theworkplacechoir.co.uk/single-post/2017/03/23/The-Gareth-Malone-Effect

6

Musical care at the end of life

Palliative care perspectives and emerging practices

Giorgos Tsiris, Jo Hockley, and Tamsin Dives

Introduction

Talking about death and dying is inevitable, and indeed vitally important, when it comes to understanding music's role in human life. The reality is that death and dying, although commonly associated with old age and illness, are of relevance across the life course. Child mortality due to illness, and death caused by war, murder, accident, or natural disasters, are only some examples that go beyond the commonly perceived 'natural progression' of life. Though aware of these multiple manifestations of death and dying in life, this chapter has a specific focus: it explores the role of musical care at, and around, the end of life, with a focus on palliative care contexts for dying adults and their communities. In this context, musical care refers to a spectrum of diverse music practices, experiences, and contexts that may range from people's everyday engagement with music, to professional, specialized music interventions.

Informed by our respective professional backgrounds, our writing embraces and promotes interdisciplinarity. We first met in 2008 while working at St Christopher's Hospice as music therapists (Giorgos and Tamsin) and a nurse consultant (Jo).[1] As members of the hospice's Arts Team, Giorgos and Tamsin developed a number of music- and arts-based health-promotion and death-education projects. Jo coordinated the St Christopher's Care Home Project Team (established in 2008) and helped lead and implement quality improvement projects in collaboration with local care homes to improve the quality of their end-of-life care provision (Kinley & Hockley, 2016). Although our respective work at St Christopher's Hospice overlapped for five years (2008–2013) and we were aware of one another's work, we did not actively collaborate. Perhaps this situation reflects many practitioners' working reality in which—partly due to workload and specialized modes of working—interdisciplinary dialogue and collaboration, beyond routine multidisciplinary meetings, are limited and often missed.

---

[1] Although Giorgos and Jo currently work in other organizations, St Christopher's Hospice is used as a shared reference point from which we draw some of the materials presented in this chapter.

Giorgos Tsiris, Jo Hockley, and Tamsin Dives, *Musical care at the end of life* In: *Collaborative Insights.* Edited by: Neta Spiro and Katie Rose M. Sanfilippo, Oxford University Press. © Oxford University Press 2022.
DOI: 10.1093/oso/9780197535011.003.0007

We argue that interdisciplinarity, as a process of integrating and applying knowledge and different ways of knowing, includes learning and relearning ways of thinking and practising across disciplines, and 'is often underpinned by different (and, at times, competing) professional vocabularies, frameworks and agendas' (Tsiris et al., 2016, p. 59; see also Spiro & Schober, 2014). In this chapter, we stretch beyond the field of music therapy to include the interdisciplinary space of music and health (Bonde, 2011) as well as perspectives from palliative care nursing. Initially, we outline the development of end-of-life care and consider its emerging continua of care between *private-public* and between *specialist-everyday* aspects of living and dying. These continua offer a conceptual framework for understanding the multifaceted nature of musical care at the end of life. We conclude by discussing future directions for interdisciplinary collaboration and research.

End-of-life care

During the early part of the 20th century, important discoveries worldwide revolutionized health care (e.g., the invention of antibiotics, X-rays, radiotherapy, chemotherapy). As a result, in the modern Western world, the hospital setting became the focus for seriously ill people who were admitted, even when cure was unlikely, in the hope that something more could be done. People with severe health care needs, including those with cancer, increasingly died in hospital with a focus on their physical needs and limited attention to other aspects of well-being.

The evolution of the hospice movement has offered a counterbalance to the aforementioned hospitalization at the end of life or what has become known as the 'medicalisation of dying' (Clark, 2005). Dame Cicely Saunders, the founder of the modern hospice movement, trained first as a nurse, next as a social worker, and then as a doctor. She advocated a holistic and interdisciplinary approach towards care at the end of life for the patient and their family. In 1967, after much campaigning and collaboration, she opened St Christopher's Hospice in South-East London—the first modern teaching and research-based hospice. It is to Saunders that the concept of 'total pain' is attributed. This concept recognizes the multidimensional nature of people's pain experience to include not only the physical domain, but also the emotional, social, and spiritual aspects of living (Baines, 1990; Clark, 2000; Saunders, 1967).

In the United Kingdom, the hospice movement became recognized as a subspecialty training area in 1987, adopting the Canadian term 'palliative care' (from the Latin *palliare,* meaning to cloak—the focus being on the person and importance of controlling symptoms rather than the disease). Hundreds of hospices have now been established around the world, with the definition of palliative care being extended from cancer to chronic diseases such as heart failure, liver disease, renal failure, and, more recently, dementia (Hockley, 2017).

Today, palliative care is commonly understood as 'the active holistic care of patients with advanced progressive illness' (The National Council for Palliative Care, 2015).

This includes management of pain and other symptoms, alongside the provision of psychological, social, and spiritual support, and regards dying as a normal process. Palliative care offers a support system not only to help patients live as actively as possible until death but also to help family members cope during the patient's illness and into bereavement.[2]

Alongside the ongoing growth of hospices, there has been increasing emphasis on quality of life and supporting people to live and die at home or in a care home and to detail their wishes in anticipation of their end-of-life care. Care home settings are arguably a vital part of palliative care—especially in relation to caring for those dying from advanced dementia. In the United Kingdom, 22% of the population dies in such settings (Laing, 2015) and this number is expected to increase to 40% by 2040 (Etkind et al., 2017).

Recognizing the importance of community involvement and of promoting healthy social attitudes towards death and dying (Kellehear, 1999), palliative care has also adopted a health-promotion and death-education role. From this perspective, palliative care's initial focus on hospice-based care of the individual patient/family has expanded over the years to embrace everyday and public aspects of living and dying (Salau et al., 2007; Sallnow et al., 2013; Stjernswärd, 2007). The emergence of compassionate communities (Kellehear, 2013) is an example of this more public and everyday face of end-of-life care. Based on a public health approach to palliative care, such communities are about 'ordinary' people providing assistance, alongside official health provision, for those in need of end-of-life care.

Emerging continua of care

Over the past decades, end-of-life care has drawn a trajectory from private and specialist palliative care practices and contexts towards more public initiatives to include everyday aspects of living and dying (Clark, 2014; Paul & Sallnow, 2013). This trajectory reflects related developments within and around the field of music therapy, too. To help conceptualize these developments and the role of musical care at the end of life, we introduce two intersecting continua between *everyday* and *specialist*, and between *public* and *private* aspects of care. In Figure 6.1 we depict these continua as well as the expansion of end-of-life care and of musical care towards public and everyday contexts of practice.

These continua of care are dynamic and depend on various factors, including the person's age, cultural context, health, and socio-economic status. On the *everyday-specialist* continuum, we understand the *everyday* to mean the commonplace or the

---

[2] There are debates regarding the distinction and relationship between 'palliative care', 'end-of-life care', and 'dying' with a range of definitions, many of which relate to the trajectory of illness progression and life expectancy (e.g., Murray et al., 2005). In this chapter, we refer to both 'palliative care' and 'end-of-life care' as pertaining to the late stage of advanced, progressive, incurable disease (often lasting a number of months). We consider 'dying' as relating to the final weeks of someone's life.

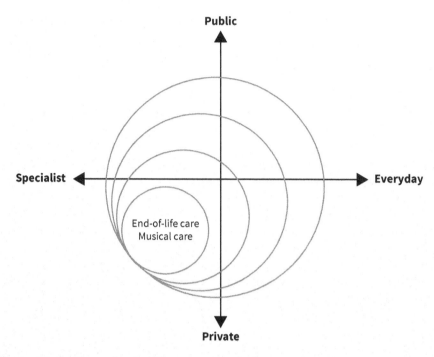

Figure 6.1 Continua of end-of-life care and musical care

daily use or activity. Conversely, *specialist* refers to in-depth, detailed knowledge or skill regarding a specific topic or area of practice and is often connected to assumptions regarding professional expertise and power. Specialist knowledge or input is typically required in 'unusual' or non-ordinary situations, such as the diagnosis of a terminal illness. On the *private-public* continuum, the *private* signifies some kind of withdrawing from public life. It is often perceived as exclusive or confidential and with a more individual focus. The concept of privacy—which is core in therapeutic professions—is interwoven with assumptions and commitments regarding ethical provision of care and research in health care. On the other hand, the *public*—which is often perceived as opposite to the private—is about openness and sharing, and commonly associated to a sense of community. These two continua as portrayed in Figure 6.1 offer a framework for exploring diverse musical care practices and their contexts in relation to care at the end of life, as we discuss in the rest of the chapter.

Musical care practices and contexts

Throughout human history, music has played a vital role in the way that people and communities have cared for the dying and for those around them. Music healing practices have been interwoven and shaped by different cultural influences, including people's spiritual beliefs regarding afterlife as well as music's divine origins and its power to connect different worlds (Gouk, 2000; Horden, 2000). In modern Western societies, a wealth of music practices, equipment, and technologies are currently available to support people in their experience of terminal illness and grief (O'Callaghan et al., 2013). Such practices range from people's everyday engagement with music to professional music interventions by professionals such as music therapists, community musicians, music thanatologists,[3] and personalized music listening specialists. Although sharing music as a common denominator, these practices vary in terms of their aims and methods, as well as their theoretical underpinnings and professional frameworks.

We first focus on music therapy, which, given its expanding practice and research base, tends to dominate the discourse around the role of music in palliative care. We then focus on musical care in relation to death education and health promotion which is commonly located within the *public* and *everyday* ends of the continua of end-of-life care (see Figure 6.1). This focus leads to an exploration of live music performance work and its role in end-of-life care, as well as an exploration of musical care by non-music professionals.

Music therapy in palliative care

End-of-life care is an important area of music therapy practice. Despite limited statutory funding for music therapy in palliative care in the United Kingdom (Graham-Wisener et al., 2018), demographic survey data suggests that end-of-life care is a growing area of music therapy work nationally and internationally (Carr et al., 2017; Kern & Tague, 2017; Silverman & Furman, 2014). Music therapy, in fact, is one of the most frequently used complementary therapies in specialist, inpatient palliative care settings in the United States (Demmer, 2004).

Music therapy in palliative care can be described as the 'creative and professionally informed use of music in a therapeutic relationship with people who are living with life-threatening illnesses, and their close family and friends' (O'Callaghan et al., 2015, p. 470). With a focus on the therapeutic relationship and process, music therapy offers a creative context to support and promote people's quality of life. This can include management of physical symptoms, psychological adjustment, emotional expression and resilience, and existential contemplation, as well as increased self-awareness and sense of well-being (O'Callaghan et al.,2015; O'Callaghan & Michael, 2017).

When reaching the end of their lives, people commonly seek creative and new ways to express themselves, to understand their current circumstances, and to come to terms with their own mortality, as well as to discover new meaning and a sense of

---

[3] Music thanatology is an emerging field within palliative care that unites music and medicine. Practitioners in the field use harp and voice at the bedside to support the dying person and their loved ones with prescriptive music (Freeman et al., 2006; Schroeder-Sheker, 1994).

hope. In the end of life, when intense emotional, psychological, and spiritual change and transformation take place, music therapy can offer a creative space for self-expression both verbal and nonverbal. The use of music improvisation, in particular, can allow and give shape and meaning to emergent forms of expression. It can offer a creative space where messy, unfinished, and unknown aspects of living and dying can be explored, articulated, and managed (Tsiris, 2018).

Creative engagement, more generally, is found to have an analgesic effect—not as a simple 'distraction' or 'diversion' but as a result of such engagement (Rawlence, 2007). Indeed, the literature suggests that music therapy is not a simple distraction but it can enable the person to refocus on their situation, change their current state of being, and promote a sense of everyday transcendence (Tsiris, 2018).

Music therapists work with terminally ill individuals as well as with their families in diverse end-of-life care settings to include hospices, day therapy centres, inpatient units, community palliative care settings, and care homes. Music therapy varies depending on the person's profile and the progression of their health condition, as well as the care context and the practitioner's own approach (O'Callaghan & Michael, 2017). Sessions can take various formats—from individual sessions to large, open, drop-in groups. Music therapy methods are commonly framed as 'active' or 'receptive'. For example, the former includes music improvisation, singing, composition, and songwriting, while the latter includes music listening and guided imagery, as well as music for relaxation and music-assisted cognitive reframing.

More specifically, the use of songs in music therapy can offer a creative and safe container—a shared music space where meanings can be discovered and expressed through metaphor and symbolism. The use of precomposed songs as well as songwriting can be a springboard for verbal reflection and personal insight that may be combined and enhanced by other creative work such as painting, writing, and movement. Analysis of lyrics written in palliative care contexts show music therapy's impact on supporting people's exploration of their current circumstances and their sense of hope, as well as its role in processing anticipatory grief (O'Callaghan, 1996; O'Callaghan et al., 2009). Therapeutic songwriting has also been used to support young adults' transition from children to adult palliative care services. Young adults' decision-making during the songwriting process—including lyrics, orchestration, and manipulation of their voice through sound effects—can offer a sense of control (Edgar et al., 2019). In and through music, people can experience such control, mastery, and self-determination that have perhaps been challenged and limited through illness. At the same time, the temporal nature of music can be a catalyst for people to experience, explore, and share their sense of change and loss. Songs and songwriting can also be an important component of life review, funeral planning, and legacy work.

Legacy work often takes the form of songs, compositions, or music-based life reviews (Hogan, 2003; O'Callaghan & Michael, 2017; O'Callaghan et al., 2009). Legacies can support both the dying individual and their families, friends and carers, supporting them to cope with loss, find meaning, and have a sense of relationship completion (Clements-Cortés, 2010). On some occasions, however, legacy work may intensify grief and distress associated with an unsatisfying relationship (Mancini et al., 2009; O'Callaghan & Michael, 2017). Legacy work often takes planning and preparation, but it can also be more spontaneous.

Family sessions can encourage creative experience for the family unit and offer a space for meaningful interaction, relationship completion, and closure (Clements-Cortés, 2018a, 2018b). Music therapy can help address anticipatory grief needs of the patient's family and their loved ones. Equally, it can facilitate the expression of grief and enhance reintegration of bereaved caregivers into their everyday lives and their communities (Krout, 2017; Magill, 2009). Research also suggests that music therapy can positively affect the interaction between people with late-stage dementia and their family caregivers. Music therapy sessions can increase people's participation, their initiation, and their responsiveness to touch with one another, as well as increase caregivers' sense of satisfaction with visits at the care setting (Clair & Ebberts, 1997).

A note on research

Research literature contains a wealth of studies exploring the role of music therapy in palliative care. A review of research publications from 1986 to 2009 demonstrates music therapy's positive impact on patients' quality of life and on families' sense of support, meaning, and empowerment (O'Callaghan, 2009). Similarly, research documents music therapy's effectiveness in reducing hospice patients' anxiety, drowsiness, pain, and tiredness (Horne-Thompson & Grocke, 2008).

Despite the breadth of the music therapy literature in palliative care, the quality of research studies in the field has been questioned (McConnell et al., 2016), especially by the evidence-based movement in which 'hard' evidence is prioritized over qualitative accounts of people's relational practices and experiences (Wigram & Gold, 2012). Based on a biomedical methodological framework, for example, a Cochrane review (Bradt & Dileo, 2010) found insufficient evidence to support the effectiveness of music therapy in palliative care. However, the review indicated that music therapy 'may have a beneficial effect on the quality of life of people in end-of-life care' (Bradt & Dileo, 2010, p. 5) and numerous single studies were identified as demonstrating: music therapy's effectiveness in terms of enhancing spirituality (Wlodarczyk, 2007); reducing tiredness and drowsiness (Horne-Thompson & Grocke, 2008); and alleviating discomfort and sadness (Nguyen, 2003). Similarly, more recent studies highlight music therapy's impact on reducing pain among palliative care patients (Gutgsell et al., 2013). A feasibility study (Porter et al., 2018) indicated improvement in terms of existential well-being, physical symptoms, and psychological support. Led by an interdisciplinary research team, this feasibility study informed the development of a treatment manual for music therapy with palliative care inpatients (Kirkwood et al., 2019).

Service evaluation findings (Gill, 2008; Graham-Wisener et al., 2018; Tsiris et al., 2014; Tsiris & Hartley, 2014) and studies exploring multidisciplinary perspectives of music therapy in end-of-life care (O'Kelly & Koffman, 2007) suggest that the impact of music therapy reaches beyond the individual dying person as well as beyond the immediate time and space where music therapy takes place. Music therapy can support relationships between clients, families, and staff. It can also enhance the broader care environment and support palliative care staff (Krout, 2017). The latter can include specialized interventions to facilitate the grief processing of health care staff who experience the deaths of patients (Popkin et al., 2011).

This distributed impact of music therapy—often described as a 'ripple effect' (Pavlicevic et al., 2015)—is supported by research findings documenting music therapy's effect on 'indirect beneficiaries' such as staff (Tsiris et al., 2020). Hilliard (2006), for example, found that team building of hospice staff improved when they either experienced free-form, improvisational music therapy, or structured sessions, including guided meditation with music. Other studies (e.g., O'Callaghan & Magill, 2009) show that staff members who witnessed music therapy on oncology wards were indirectly supported by the sessions and felt that their patient care had improved. Improved staff mood and resilience are also documented in the literature (McConnell et al., 2016; O'Kelly & Koffman, 2007).

Ethnographic studies of music therapy in hospice and care home settings (as discussed in the Musical care in older adulthood chapter and, e.g., Tsiris, 2018; Wood, 2015) show that music therapists perceive their role as working with the whole organization. They see music therapy, and music more broadly, as contributing to the overall organizational well-being to include not only those who are referred to the music therapy service, but also those who are, directly or indirectly, part of the music-making ecology. Often ranging from community-oriented work, to live performance and coordination of hospice music events, such practices offer some kind of 'invisible care' to the whole organization and its community, affecting the soundscapes and people's experiences of the care environment (Tsiris, 2018).

Interdisciplinary collaboration

Music therapists collaborate closely with other palliative care professionals contributing to holistic care and treatment planning (Krout, 2004), but interdisciplinary approaches to music therapy practice and research in the field are scarcely documented. Slivka and Magilld (1986), for example, report the provision of conjoint family sessions with social worker and music therapist to support communication, through songwriting, between children and parents when one of the parents was dying. Magill and Berenson (2008) write about the conjoint use of music therapy and reflexology with hospitalized advanced-stage cancer patients and their families. Anecdotal information indicates further examples such as the use of music therapy to support physiotherapy for well-being classes, the provision of live and recorded music to help patients relax and cope with palliative radiography, and collaboration between music therapists, pastoral, and spiritual care professionals (e.g., Haghighi & Pansch, 2000; Krout, 2017; O'Callaghan et al., 2015).

Furthermore, music therapists often collaborate with other music and arts practitioners, such as performing art therapies, community artists, and musicians (Hartley, 2008, 2014). Curtis (2011) reports a collaborative project between a university music therapy training program, a professional symphony orchestra, and a regional hospital in Canada. The project included 371 adult patients over a three-year period in an in-patient palliative care unit. The results showed that patients experienced pain relief and relaxation, as well as an enhanced sense of quality of life.

Interdisciplinary collaboration between music therapists and other music and arts practitioners in palliative care is scarcely documented in the literature (e.g., Shoemark, 2009). Despite the sceptical engagement of music therapists with the wider 'arts in health' movement (Hartley, 2008), such interdisciplinary work has the potential to enrich practice development as well as expand methodological approaches to musical care. In recent years, there seems to be an increased opportunity for such collaborative work often relating to public and everyday domains of end-of-life care (see Figure 6.1) and with specific reference to death-education and health-promotion initiatives, as will be discussed.

Music's role in death-education and health-promoting palliative care

Living and dying are often perceived as two opposite ends of a spectrum. Death is often perceived as an unwelcome guest and a threat to our well-being. It is regarded as a failure of medicine and our technologically advanced society. Despite positive changes that have taken place in terms of influencing professionals' attitudes towards death and dying, and improving care for the dying, there has been little shift in public perception. Death and dying remain a taboo.

Society's focus on technological advancement and technical solutions to the inevitability of ageing and death has dramatic consequences to our subjective and collective experience of death and grief, with terminally ill people experiencing a kind of social death, hopelessness, and dismay (Monroe, 2014). Changing this death-denying culture and promoting public conversation about death, loss, and grief have now become key priorities in end-of-life care policy and practice within and beyond the United Kingdom (Department of Health, 2008). In response, numerous community-oriented and intergenerational musical care initiatives have emerged with a focus on everyday and public aspects of care (see Figure 6.1). We will explore such initiatives by drawing on examples from our practice experience at St Christopher's Hospice in London and at St Columba's Hospice Care in Edinburgh, respectively.

Community-oriented musical care

Music, and the arts more generally, have emerged as catalysts in enabling hospices to engage with their local communities and in disrupting societal taboos around death and dying. In diverse forms, formats, and media, ranging from one-off performances to long-term projects, the arts can bring people together in creative and non-threatening ways (All-Party Parliamentary Group on Arts, Health and Wellbeing, 2017; Bertman, 2018; Hartley, 2011, 2014). With diverse applications in palliative and bereavement care, music and songwriting in particular can be a powerful way to express, articulate, and share experiences of loss and change as well as to change perception and to build emotional resilience and social bonding (Heath & Lings, 2012; Tsiris et al., 2011). By opening up hospitable, creative, and reflective spaces, music and the arts allow individuals to share difficult experiences and topics with others, to seek support and understanding, and help them to integrate healthily and creatively death and dying into their everyday lives. The community choir at St Christopher's Hospice is an example of a community-oriented musical care initiative underpinned by a public health approach to palliative care.

Community choir

In 2011, Tamsin and Giorgos established the community choir at St Christopher's Hospice as part of a wider social programme aiming to welcome the general public into the hospice, offering a positive experience and a different perspective of 'hospice life'. The choir, which has been led by Tamsin since 2015, is open to anyone and includes a mixture of patients, volunteers, staff, and bereaved family members from the local community. Since its establishment, the choir has slowly grown and now numbers over 100. The choir meets in the central public space of the hospice building, where patients and visiting family often have supper and a cup of tea. Music by its very nature can invade spaces, demanding attention. It has few constrictions and porous boundaries, offering hospitable and welcoming spaces for people to be together. Each Monday evening the singing ripples through the building and connects patients, visitors, and staff. The choir brings the ordinariness of daily life into the hospice. It also attracts some of the more isolated members of the local community into a place of warmth and friendship. In singing together, for a brief moment patient, nurse, mourner, and volunteer are side by side. Coming together to sing offers a place of comfort, a space to personally reflect. Through its performances within and beyond the hospice premises (Photograph 6.1), the choir has also become a vehicle to communicate the hospice's values and ethos to the wider public.

Feedback from choir members highlight its impact on health promotion and death education:

I find being in the choir is a lovely experience. It is a good idea to rehearse in the café area, as it appears to bring solace to the relatives visiting their loved ones at a difficult time. The experience has changed my ideas about what a hospice might be.

Singing in the choir at St Christopher's has been a joyful experience; to share the making of music and singing with others of all ages and backgrounds. I have found it to be encouraging to experience the enjoyment and participation of those who are having treatments in the hospice, and relatives and friends who visit; to witness how people can benefit from joining in the creative experience, by watching, listening,

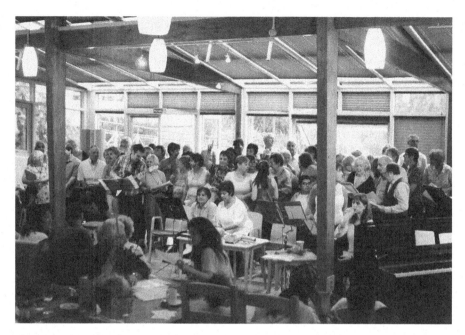

Photograph 6.1 Performance of the community choir at St Christopher's Hospice

and sometimes singing engenders a sense of well-being and of 'no walls between'
death, dying, and the ongoing creative activities of life.

Such community-oriented work highlights how music can bring people together, create new communities, and function as an agent for social transformation. The preceding example shows how a community choir can generate a space within which a diverse mix of people come together to sing and, on many occasions, to share (more or less openly), their narratives of living and dying. Through such community choir work, a sense of respect for one another and their contributions as fellow musicians, beyond health-illness and professional identities, is fostered. The community choir can become a microcosm where all involved have opportunities to learn and relearn new skills as well as change their attitudes towards living and dying. Community choirs can relocate death and dying as a natural part of community life, changing the hospice's image as a more everyday and less medicalized and isolated environment (Tsiris, 2018). The success of such community-oriented work—given its whole organization and systemic approach—often depends on interdisciplinarity collaboration and investment involving clinical, administrative, and managerial areas of the hospice life.

Intergenerational musical care

The recognition that children and young people are catalysts in any sustainable social change has led to the development of intergenerational projects as another important area of public approaches to palliative care, including death education. Working with children and schools is crucial not only for shaping healthier attitudes towards death and dying, but also for raising childhood grief awareness and equipping school communities to support children in their own experiences of change, loss, and transition in life. This support seems particularly important, considering that in the United Kingdom, for example, around 111 children are bereaved of a parent every day (Child Bereavement UK, 2017).

> **Change matters**
> In 2019, as part of its expanding community engagement and health-promotion work, the Arts and the Family Support services of St Columba's Hospice Care in collaboration with Fischy Music, a community music organization, implemented an intergenerational project. Hospice patients and children from a local primary school were brought together to explore, express, and share through music their experiences of grief, change, and loss in life. This short-term project included school-wide input for both students and staff. It involved music workshops on 'Hellos' and 'Goodbyes' with a focus on emotional well-being, staff training on childhood loss and bereavement, and how to support all this in the school setting, as well as more focused songwriting work with a group of 10 P5–6 children. The resulting song, which was titled 'Change Matters', was recorded and also performed at a closing event at the hospice. This was an open event attracting children's families as well as members of the public and drew media attention.

This project enabled children to talk openly about death and dying, and taking a whole-school approach, it also equipped school staff with confidence and skills (St Columba's Hospice Care, 2020; Tsiris et al., 2019).

> You don't really have to be afraid of maybe talking to someone about your worries ... Change matters; it's not something that you have to hide. (Child)
>   I will introduce it [loss] as a subject that should be talked about and tell the class it's OK to talk about it. (School staff)
>   Many still consider death a taboo subject for children but it is vital that we talk to children about death. Most children will be affected by the death of someone in their family or family friends and they need to know what this means practically and how to deal with this emotionally, too. We enjoyed performing our songs and developing resources for schools across the city to share. (Head teacher)

Similar projects have taken place in many hospices. Notably, St Christopher's Hospice has led numerous music- and arts-based intergenerational projects. Since 2005, these projects have brought to the hospice diverse school communities, including students from local special-needs schools, and four key evaluation themes have emerged: changing attitudes towards living and dying; normalizing death and dying; patients as educators; and, creating and sustaining healthy relationships (Hartley, 2011; Tsiris et al., 2011).

'Soundtracks' is an example of an intergenerational project bringing together teenagers, patients, and carers between St Christopher's Hospice and the BRIT School for Performing Arts & Technology in South-East London.

Soundtracks

Over a period of eight weeks, hospice patients and BRIT School students are partnered with the purpose of writing, performing, and recording songs together. Patients share their stories and biographies identifying together with the students the emerging song themes. Students are challenged to compose music and write about things they might not usually explore, such as illness and transition in life. Patients are invited to talk about matters they would not usually share with younger people. The songs that emerge as a result of bringing these two groups of people together are often surprising and powerful. The project ends with a public performance that is open to everyone, including patients' and students' families and friends, as well as the hospice and school staff members. Based on feedback over the years, 'Soundtracks' provides both patients and students with new experiences (Photograph 6.2). For the students, it brings them into a palliative care environment in a non-threatening way. It 'stretches' them creatively and develops their emotional literacy. Patients and carers, many of whom are socially and emotionally isolated through dealing with terminal illness, often relish the chance to engage with younger people, to tell their story, to have it witnessed, acknowledged, and celebrated.

Community-oriented musical care and intergenerational work can challenge assumptions and expand perceptions of patients as 'care receivers' and of professionals as 'caregivers'. Such work can empower communities and enable individuals to meet one another on an equal basis and reintegrate with their local community. It can also generate new images of hospice care and highlight new possibilities for inter- and transdisciplinary working. This includes repositioning hospices as resource hubs for their local communities by fostering partnerships and opportunities for open dialogue and creative action around death, dying, change, and loss.

Live music performance

Live music performance is another important area of musical care in end-of-life care with diverse applications across the *everyday-specialist* and *private-public* continua (see Figure 6.1). Playing live music to people who are terminally ill has been important since the early practice of music as therapy back in the 1970s (Munro & Mount,

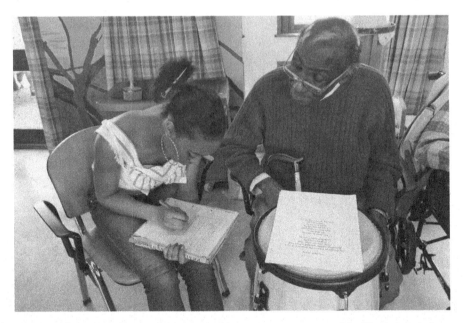

Photograph 6.2 Student and patient working on a song as part of the 'Soundtracks' project

1978). This includes accompanying someone during the last moments of their life. In recent years, however, there has been an increased interest in the role of live music performances and concerts within hospices and care homes. The scope and format of such performances can vary significantly to include, for example, ticketed concerts and more ad hoc performances, as well as the rise of initiatives such as dementia-friendly concerts and the Threshold Choir in the United States—a group dedicated to live singing for those at the threshold of life.

Performance-oriented musical care draws on a growing recognition of the role of music and more generally of the arts in addressing the aesthetic deprivation of people in health care settings (Canga et al., 2012; Moss, 2014). Music and the arts can foster a creative environment and a place to die with dignity (NHS Estates Design Brief Working Group, 2005; Waller & Finn, 2011). Studies from the field of arts and health and beyond (e.g., Moss et al., 2007) demonstrate the impact of live music on transforming the care environment, and in recent years numerous initiatives have grown, bringing performing musicians to health care settings. Such initiatives aim to bring music to patients who may have little, if any, access to live music and to improve quality of life for patients, their families, and staff.

Evaluation data shows that live music in hospital (e.g., Moss et al., 2007), as also discussed in the Musical care in older adulthood chapter, enhances the quality of the aesthetic environment of the hospital, with both patients and staff stating that listening to live music helped them to relax and feel happier and more positive. Music was found to have strong emotional effect, while patients' perception of the hospital was affected positively by live music in waiting areas. Drawing on their education and psychology backgrounds, Marshall and Shibazaki (2016) studied how musical concerts can contribute to the well-being of all those involved in end-of-life care contexts. Results deriving from observations and interviews with patients, family members, and staff who experienced a musical event show that people's experience of live music offered emotional support, promoting new and positive memories, and provided brief periods of respite for all those involved. They found that live music concerts contributed to the creation of 'asylum' (a term used by music sociologist Tia DeNora [2013] describing music's capacity to generate a 'space' for respite, care, and a new sense of self) for the clients, the families, and the nursing and care staff. Marshall and Shibazaki argue that music concerts can offer respite from distress and pain, and can promote a sense of 'flow' and creativity. For some patients, the concerts also offered a creative and meaningful experience that they could share together with their visiting families.

In addition to the live music work offered by organizations such as the United Kingdom's Live Music Now, and Music in Hospitals and Care, many live music initiatives are organized more locally, often by the music therapist onsite. The discourse and practice of community music therapy has also fuelled a renewed interest in music therapy as an ecological practice (Stige et al., 2010) and music therapists' role in 'the promotion of health within and between various layers of the sociocultural community and/or physical environment' (Schmid, 2018, p.147). Following are two examples of live music initiatives at St Columba's Hospice and St Christopher's Hospice Care, respectively.

Iona Music

Giorgos has developed 'Iona Music'—a live music performance programme at St Columba's Hospice Care (see Photograph 6.3). Musicians from the local community are invited to perform at Iona Café, which is the social hub of the hospice. These performances are open to patients and families, as well as to the public. In addition to changing the hospice environment, such performance-oriented work opens up the hospice doors to the local community and transforms perceptions around what a hospice is, or what it can be about. Many of these musicians would not normally perform to a hospice care environment and this work invites them to adopt an informal musical care role. Some musicians are connected to the hospice through personal experience of loss and for some offering live music is a way to reconnect with the hospice.

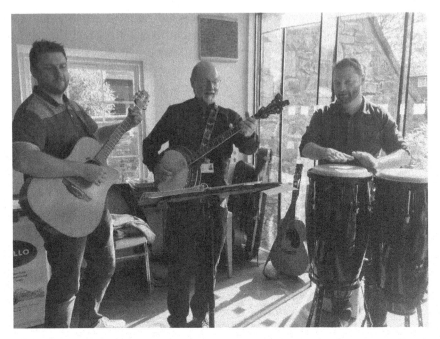

Photograph 6.3 Local musicians playing at St Columba's Hospice Care

---

Cicely Saunders Concert Series

Tamsin has led the development of the Cicely Saunders Concert Series at St Christopher's Hospice. Inviting professional and often well-known musicians at the hospice, this monthly Concert Series has focused on welcoming the public into the hospice and promoting healthier attitudes towards death and dying. The diverse range of the programme—from acoustic folk, to string quartets, to Indian and rock music—reflects the demographic of the surrounding area and people's cultural diversity. The audience combines local community members together with staff, patients, and their families. Completing its tenth year, the series has welcomed hundreds of members of the general public and has had a huge impact on the hospice's integration with its local community.

Such performance work, as illustrated in the two preceding examples, highlights the more public applications of musical care and its possibilities when brought within specialist palliative care environments (see Figure 6.1). Many of the visiting musicians remark they have never felt so listened to. Performing in a hospice setting transforms their experience of playing music. Perhaps the combination of the local audience and those facing the ends of their lives facilitates a particular quality of attention, of listening and togetherness at these concerts. Music promotes remembrance, reflection, and recollection, and, it is particularly so at these events.

Indeed, ethnographic music therapy research shows that live music concerts within a hospice environment can reawaken people's quest for meaning, connection, and change, and can remind them of their own mortality (Tsiris, 2018). Such performance work can transform the hospice into a concert venue; it highlights other possibilities for community engagement and invites us to reimagine the hospice as a resource for the broader community beyond caring for the dying. Equally, results from care home settings show that live music can change the cultural environment of the care home and the behaviour of the residents. Live music's ripple effect can transform the atmosphere, lifting the mood of the residents and care staff alike and generating a sense of connectedness (Pavlicevic et al., 2015; Tapson et al., 2018).

Musical care by non-music professionals

Within health and social care contexts, musical care is typically associated with the work of music experts or 'specialists' such as music therapists, community musicians, and music performers. Research (DeNora, 2000; Gabrielsson, 2010), however, sheds light on *everyday* uses of music and informal music practices, often in the absence of specialists (as discussed in Musical care in adulthood chapter). Examples include the use of a personal listening device while one is exercising, singing when one is in the shower, and the use of music in funerals or as a form of musical self-care. Despite their relevance across the lifespan, such everyday, informal music practices remain largely undocumented in palliative care, wherein the focus tends to be on music therapy practice.

Musical care in the end of life includes one's own use of music for self-care (a concept also discussed in the Musical care in adulthood and Musical care in older adulthood chapters), often in the form of music listening. Listening to music can help people understand, regulate, and express emotions associated with pain, loss, and grief. Music can evoke and strengthen positive emotions, but it can also intensify and prolong difficult emotions (Gabrielsson, 2010; Juslin & Laukka, 2004; Skånland, 2012). DeNora (2012) found that music is often used to recall people they cared about, to remember the absent or deceased. Vist and Bonde (2013), for example, explore the affordances of music listening in relation to a parent's grieving process following the loss of a child. This includes experiencing music as comfort and consolation, offering catharsis and building resilience. Stimulating discussion about life memories, music listening can support reflection on past, present and future, and generate a sense of remembrance, connectedness, and hope (Krout, 2017).

DeNora (2012) proposes an ecological perspective for music in the end-of-life context taking account of the temporal-cultural complexity of death and dying. Using the example of everyday musical interaction in a domestic context of death and dying, she explores how musical praxis can illuminate the cultural and situational figuration of end-of-life experience both for the dying individual and the social microcosm around them. Wellness and illness are seen as inextricably linked, and music can be a dynamic medium for collective performances of meaning in living and dying.

Such ecological and community perspectives shed light on people's everyday engagement with music, a focus of the Musical care in adulthood chapter, but also highlight new professionalization trajectories for music specialists. New roles for music therapists have emerged in terms of equipping non-music specialists to engage with musical care practices in their everyday practice. Music therapists can play an important role in developing such skills and awareness to other health care staff and to family carers; to support clients, but also to consider how music can be utilized as self-care in everyday life.

Keeping Relationships Alive

Keeping Relationships Alive was a project, funded by the St James foundation and facilitated by music therapists at St Christopher's Hospice. The project aimed to explore how personal relationships with music could become a valuable resource for the caregiver and address psychosocial challenges faced by people with advanced dementia at the end of life and their informal carers. Participants were encouraged to use music with special associations as a form of caring, offering different ways for carer and patient to be together. Music can awaken qualities in people in the final stages of dementia. There is the possibility of emotional connection and intimacy at a time when communication is becoming more challenging. Music as a form of leisure can be a way of sharing time together. The music therapists shared simple skills from their musical toolkit to encourage caregivers to actively engage in music. Simple activities such as turn-taking, enjoying rhythmic games, singing, and listening to music together offered possibilities for shared activities and ones that could be patient-led. A daughter was moved to tears to realize that her elderly dying mother was making choices about how she played a tambourine—the simplest of tiny movements, yet colourful and individual.

Musical care for carers is an example of an emerging emphasis in equipping and empowering people to use music for well-being, for their own self-care. Other initiatives, such as Playlist for Life, have attracted public attention and offered a framework for non-music professionals to help people to engage with music listening for well-being purposes (Donaldson et al., 2019). Despite the scepticism that such initiatives have faced, they have grown and are currently applied in diverse contexts, with care homes being a prominent example. Archie et al. (2013) stress that the role of music listening in palliative care may be underestimated. They argue that music listening, whether experienced, for example, in the form of a playlist on a portable device with headphones or live music by a music therapist or other music practitioner, can offer a sense of reassurance and familiarity across a person's disease trajectory.

Jo coordinated the St Christopher's Care Home Project Team (2008–2013) and helped lead and implement quality improvement projects in collaboration with local care homes to improve the quality of their end-of-life care provision. One of the projects included implementing the Namaste Care programme (Simard, 2014; Stacpoole et al., 2015; Stacpoole et al., 2017) to enhance and enrich, through daily sensory input, the quality of life for people with advanced dementia. Designed to stimulate the five senses, this programme is an example in which care staff, who may or may not have any formal music training, integrate music as part of their care provision. Musical care at the end of life has a role in stimulating musical memories, especially in advanced dementia where the ability to communicate has been lost, as was also discussed in the chapter on Musical care in older adulthood. On one occasion music being played by care staff during a Namaste Care session helped staff understand a patient in a new light and so transform their own responses.

Italian aria

The morning Namaste Care session had been going for an hour or so. Suddenly, Rosa [pseudonym], a resident with moderately advanced dementia, walked into the lounge and pulled aside the curtained-off area to join the session where an Italian aria CD was being played. Rosa generally found it difficult to settle and normally spent her time wandering from room to room in a somewhat agitated state. To the staff's utter amazement, Rosa started singing along in Italian. She not only sang beautifully but her singing was also word perfect. The staff were stunned. None of them had any idea that Rosa had such a lovely voice and could sing in Italian. No longer was she known as the irritated resident whom everyone needed to take a wide berth around but Rosa with the beautiful voice—through the Italian aria, staff's respect for Rosa changed. Something of who Rosa was had been revealed through the aria. The music had stimulated memories long gone, bringing her pleasure and at the same time transforming people's response to her.

As highlighted by this account, as well as similar accounts in the literature (e.g., Peng, 2018), music taps into and brings to the fore our shared humanity. People's engagement with music when they are faced with a terminal illness can be transformational for them as well as for the people around them. The person can be seen in a different light—a creative human being who can flourish until the very end of their life. Music can humanize our understanding of people and of the care environment.

Future directions

Despite the wealth of musical care practices in end-of-life care, the literature to date has focused on music therapy work and its impact on dying individuals and their families. Research is commonly conducted by music therapists focusing on music therapy work; most involve hospice settings, with only a few studies exploring home-based or other end-of-life care contexts (Schmid & Ostermann, 2010).

We argue that future research needs to pay greater attention to the context within which musical care work takes place to acknowledge cultural and organizational dynamics. It also needs to acknowledge and document musical care in relation to community engagement and health promotion work, and to encompass practices beyond the field of music therapy. All this includes musical care provided by music specialists such as community musicians and performing musicians, as well as non-music specialists such as other health and social care staff. It also includes everyday uses of music by patients, families, and carers themselves without the presence of a professional.

There is a need to expand and diversify the current research endeavours pertaining to music therapy and other musical care practices, especially those which are rarely documented and generally remain under-researched. To this end, interdisciplinary dialogue and collaboration are crucial, allowing a synthesis of approaches that ensures both the maintenance and mutual enriching of multiple practices, theoretical perspectives, and professional frameworks (Jensenius, 2012; Stember, 1991; Tsiris et al., 2016). Such interdisciplinary dialogue needs to include both different music-based disciplines and collaboration with other fields, such as nursing and spiritual care. Archie et al. (2013), for example, call for greater collaboration between music therapy and music neuroscience in palliative care. Such collaboration may also shed light on the potential role of music at different stages of illness trajectory and progression.

We also need to diversify our methods to include service evaluation and arts-based methodologies. Our methods should prioritize and promote user involvement by engaging with the people who make the hospice community, including patients, their families, staff, and the local community. By understanding what matters to them, we will enrich current understandings of the role of music at the end of life. For example, a potential mismatch between patients and health care providers' understanding of music therapy's impact has been observed. Professionals tend to focus on the measurement of symptoms such as pain and anxiety, whereas patients and families focus on the promotion of well-being and on music therapy's impact on the improvement or completion of their relationships (Schmid, 2018; Schmid et al., 2018).

Despite the growth of the research literature, music therapy assessment in palliative care remains a relatively undocumented area. Maue-Johnson and Tanguay (2006) identified three published music therapy assessment tools, including their own, the 'Hospice Music Therapy Assessment', which aims to identify current level of functioning and to obtain information required for formulating an appropriate care plan. The lack of published tools suggests there are challenges in formulating an appropriate assessment tool to be used in hospice music therapy.

Research and evaluation in palliative care present an array of ethical dilemmas and challenges that can lead to the limited representation of dying people's voices in the literature (Haraldsdottir et al., 2019). There is a need for a greater representation and involvement of dying people in our research endeavours. An example is consideration of ethical dilemmas posed to the randomization of dying patients and the sensitivity required for collecting data from dying patients and their caregivers (McWhinney et al., 1994). Haraldsdottir et al. (2019) stress the need for a relational approach to research and research ethics in palliative care. Striking a balance between research ideals, real-life conditions, and practice ethics is of essence. Some of the challenges around randomization in palliative care were carefully considered in the MusiQual study ascertaining the feasibility of carrying out a larger multicentre trial into the effectiveness of music therapy in improving the quality of life of palliative care inpatients (Kirkwood et al., 2020).

Schmid (2018) proposes a conceptual framework for community-based participatory music therapy research in end-of-life care scenarios. He puts forward an integrative design for participatory research and the idea to meet with collaboration the complexities specific to research in end-of-life care. To this end, participatory and action-oriented approaches can offer useful methodological frameworks (Hockley et al., 2013; Stige, 2005) wherein context-responsive research questions emerge. Debates about different research methodologies are ongoing, with some authors stressing the need for validated outcome measures in routine practice (Graham-Wisener et al., 2018) and with others prioritizing the development of bespoke evaluation tools that are practice- and context-responsive.

As we have discussed in this chapter, drawing from the literature and our respective professional experiences as music therapists and a specialist nurse, musical care at the end of life can take diverse forms characterized by varying aims, practices, and contexts. We discussed these diverse forms while considering the *private-public* and *specialist-everyday* continua of musical care at the end of life. A common denominator across all forms of musical care is music's ability to reach and support people across their health-illness trajectories. Musical care can offer a sense of well-being and promote quality of life for the dying person and those around them, including their family as well as the broader community within which the care setting is located. It can generate a sense of individual as well as communal flourishing by encompassing the interconnections between people and their environments. Musical care can transform the end-of-life care environment and offer a generous space where the unknowns, tensions, and resolutions of living and dying can be embraced, expressed, and celebrated.

Acknowledgements

We would like to thank Dr Wolfgang Schmid, Professor in Music Therapy (University of Bergen, Norway) and Music Therapist (Sunniva Centre for Palliative Care, Haraldsplass Deaconess Hospital, Norway), and Dr Barry Laird, Senior Lecturer in Palliative Medicine (University of Edinburgh, United Kingdom) and Consultant in

Palliative Medicine (St Columba's Hospice Care, United Kingdom) for commenting on earlier versions of this chapter.

References

All-Party Parliamentary Group on Arts, Health and Wellbeing. (2017). *Creative health: The arts for health and wellbeing.* https://www.culturehealthandwellbeing.org.uk/appg-inquiry/

Archie, P., Bruera, E., & Cohen, L. (2013). Music-based interventions in palliative cancer care: A review of quantitative studies and neurobiological literature. *Supportive Care in Cancer, 21*(9), 2609–2624.

Baines, M. (1990). Tackling total pain. In C. Saunders (Ed.), *Hospice and palliative care: An interdisciplinary approach.* Edward Arnold.

Bertman, S. L. (2018). *Grief and the healing arts: Creativity as therapy.* Routledge.

Bonde, L. O. (2011). Health musicing—Music therapy or music and health? A model, empirical examples and personal reflections. *Music and Arts in Action, 3*(2), 120–140.

Bradt, L., & Dileo, C. (2010). Music therapy for end-of-life care. *Cochrane Database of Systematic Reviews, 2010*(1), CD007169.

Canga, B., Hahm, C. L., Lucido, D., Grossbard, M. L., & Loewy, J. V. (2012). Environmental music therapy: A pilot study on the effects of music therapy in a chemotherapy infusion suite. *Music and Medicine, 4*(4), 221–230.

Carr, C. E., Tsiris, G., & Swijghuisen Reigersberg, M. (2017). Understanding the present, re-visioning the future: An initial mapping of music therapists in the United Kingdom. *British Journal of Music Therapy, 31*(2), 68–85.

Child Bereavement UK. (2017). UK Death and Berevement Statistics. Office for National Statistics; National Records of Scotland; Northern Ireland Statistics and Research Agency.

Clair, A. A., & Ebberts, A. G. (1997). The effects of music therapy on interactions between family caregivers and their care receivers with late stage dementia. *Journal of Music Therapy, 34*(3), 148–164. https://doi.org/10.1093/jmt/34.3.148

Clark, D. (2000). Total pain: The work of Cicely Saunders and the hospice movement. *American Pain Society Bulletin, 10*(4), 13–15.

Clark, D. (2005). Cicely Saunders—Founder of the hospice movement: Selected letters 1959–1999. Oxford University Press.

Clark, D. (2014). 'Total pain': The work of Cicely Saunders and the maturing of a concept. http://endoflifestudies.academicblogs.co.uk/total-pain-the-work-of-cicely-saunders-and-the-maturing-of-a-concept/

Clements-Cortés, A. (2010). The role of music therapy in facilitating relationship completion in end-of-life care. *Canadian Journal of Music Therapy, 16*(1), 123–147.

Clements-Cortés, A. (2018a). Relationship completion in palliative care music therapy: Clinical case example—Part 1. *Music and Medicine, 10*(2), 80–90.

Clements-Cortés, A. (2018b). Relationship completion in palliative care music therapy: Clinical case research overview and results—Part 2. *Music and Medicine, 10*(2), 91–97.

Curtis, S. L. (2011). Music therapy and the symphony: A university-community collaborative project in palliative care. *Music and Medicine, 3*(1), 20–26.

Demmer, C. (2004). A survey of complementary therapy services provided by hospices. *Journal of Palliative Medicine, 7*(4), 510–516.

DeNora, T. (2000). *Music in everyday life.* Cambridge: Cambridge University Press.

DeNora, T. (2012). Resounding the great divide: Theorising music in everyday life at the end of life. *Mortality, 17*(2), 92–105.

DeNora, T. (2013). *Music asylums: Wellbeing through music in everyday life.* Ashgate.

Department of Health (2008). *End of life care strategy: Promoting high quality care for all adults at the end of life.*

Donaldson, K., McLean, J., Collins, L., Cruickshank, F., & Haraldsdottir, E. (2019). Music to my ears: Implementing personalised music playlists in a hospice inpatient unit (IPU). *BMJ Supportive & Palliative Care, 9*(Suppl.4), A64.

Edgar, J., Tsiris, G., & Rickson, D. (2019). 'The screams crashed into silence': A therapeutic songwriting project for young adults with life-shortening illnesses. In A. Ludwig (Ed.), *Music therapy in children's palliative care* (pp. 159–173). Jessica Kingsley Publishers.

Etkind, S. N., Bone, A. E., Gomes, B., Lovell, N., Evans, C. J., Higginson, I. J., & Murtagh, F. E. M. (2017). How many people will need palliative care in 2040? Past trends, future projections and implications for services. *BMC Medicine, 15*(1), 102.

Freeman, L., Caserta, M., Lund, D., Rossa, S., Dowdy, A., & Partenheimer, A. (2006). Music thanatology: Prescriptive harp music as palliative care for the dying patient. *American Journal of Hospice and Palliative Medicine, 23*(2), 100–104.

Gabrielsson, A. (2010). *Strong experiences with music.* Oxford University Press.

Gill, A. (2008). Music and music therapy at St Christopher's Hospice–An evaluation study. In N. Hartley & M. Payne (Eds.), *The creative arts in palliative care* (pp. 172–185). Jessica Kingsley Publishers.

Gouk, P. (Ed.). (2000). *Musical healing in cultural contexts.* Ashgate.

Graham-Wisener, L., Watts, G., Kirkwood, J., Harrison, C., McEwan, J., Porter, S., Reid, J., & McConnell, T. (2018). Music therapy in UK palliative and end-of-life care: A service evaluation. *BMJ Supportive & Palliative Care, 8*(3), 282–284.

Gutgsell, K. J., Schluchter, M., & Margevicius, S. (2013). Music therapy reduces pain in palliative care patients: A randomized controlled trial. *Journal of Pain and Symptom Management, 45,* 822–831.

Haraldsdottir, E., Lloyd, A., & Dewing, J. (2019). Relational ethics in palliative care research: Including a person-centred approach. *Palliative Care and Social Practice, 13,* 1–7.

Hartley, N. (2008). The arts in health and social care—Is music therapy fit for purpose? *British Journal of Music Therapy, 22*(2), 88–96.

Hartley, N. (2011). Letting it out of the cage: Death education and community involvement. In S. Conway (Ed.), *Governing death and loss—Empowerment, involvement and participation* (pp. 129–137). Oxford University Press.

Hartley, N. (Ed.). (2014). *End of life care: A guide for therapists, artists and arts therapists.* Jessica Kingsley Publishers.

Heath, B., & Lings, J. (2012). Creative songwriting in therapy at the end of life and in bereavement. *Mortality, 17*(2), 106–118.

Hilliard, R. (2006). The effect of music therapy sessions on compassion fatigue and team building of professional hospice caregivers. *Arts in Psychotherapy, 33,* 395–401.

Hockley, J., Froggat, K., & Heimerl, K. (Eds.). (2013). *Participatory research in palliative care: Actions and reflections.* Oxford University Press.

Hockley, J. (2017). Hospices and care homes—similarities and differences in relation to palliative care. *Annals of Palliative Medicine, 6*(4), 396–398.

Hogan, B. E. (2003). Soul music in the twilight years: Music therapy and the dying process. *Topics in Geriatric Rehabilitation, 19*(4), 275–281.

Horden, P. (Ed.). (2000). *Music as medicine: The history of music therapy since antiquity.* Ashgate.

Horne-Thompson, A., & Grocke, D. (2008). The effect of music therapy on anxiety in patients who are terminally ill. *Journal of Palliative Medicine, 11*(4), 582–590.

Jensenius, A. R. (2012). *Disciplinarities: Intra, cross, multi, inter, trans.* http://www.arj.no/2012/03/12/disciplinarities-2/

Juslin, P. N., & Laukka, P. (2004). Expression, perception, and induction of musical emotions: A review and a questionnaire study of everyday listening. *Journal of New Music Research*, *33*(3), 217–238.

Kellehear, A. (1999). *Health promoting palliative care*. Oxford University Press.

Kellehear, A. (2013). Compassionate communities: End-of-life care as everyone's responsibility. *QJM: An International Journal of Medicine*, *106*(12), 1071–1075.

Kern, P., & Tague, D. B. (2017). Music therapy practice status and trends worldwide: An international survey study. *Journal of Music Therapy*, *54*(3), 255–286.

Kinley, J., & Hockley, J. (2016). A practice development initiative supporting care home staff deliver high quality end of life care. *International Journal of Palliative Nursing*, *22*(10), 474–481.

Kirkwood, J., Graham-Wisener, L., McConnell, T., Porter, S., Reid, J., Craig, N., Dunlop, C., Gordon, C., Thomas, D., Godsal, J., & Vorster, A. (2019). The MusiQual treatment manual for music therapy in a palliative care inpatient setting. *British Journal of Music Therapy*, *33*(1), 5–15.

Kirkwood, J., Graham-Wisener, L., McConnell, T., Porter, S., & Reid, J. (2020). A synopsis of the MusiQual feasibility study into the effectiveness of music therapy in palliative care inpatient settings. *Approaches: An Interdisciplinary Journal of Music Therapy*, *12*(2), 171–184.

Krout, R. E. (2004). A synerdisciplinary music therapy treatment team approach for hospice and palliative care. *Australian Journal of Music Therapy*, *15*, 33–45.

Haghighi, K. R., & Pansch, B. (2000). Music therapy. In National Hospice and Palliative Care Organization (Ed.), *Complementary therapies in end-of-life care* (pp. 53–68). Alexandria, VA: National Hospice and Palliative Care Organization.

Krout, R. E. (2017). Music therapy for grief and loss. In B. Wheeler (Ed.), *Music therapy handbook* (pp. 401–411). Guilford Press.

Laing, W. (2015). *Care of older people—UK market report* (27th ed.). Laing & Buisson.

Magill, L. (2009). Caregiver empowerment and music therapy: Through the eyes of bereaved caregivers of advanced cancer patients. *Journal of Palliative Care*, *25*(1), 68–75.

Mancini, A. D., Robinaugh, D., Shear, K., & Bonanno, G. A. (2009). Does attachment avoidance help people cope with loss? The moderating effects of relationship quality. *Journal of Clinical Psychology*, *65*(10), 1127–1136.

Marshall, N. A., & Shibazaki, K. (2016). Seeking asylum: The benefits for clients, family members and care-givers of using music in hospice care. *Asian Journal of Human Services*, *11*, 18–30.

McConnell, T., Scott, D., & Porter, S. (2016). Music therapy for end-of-life care: An updated systematic review. *Palliative Medicine*, *30*(9), 877–883.

McWhinney, I. R., Bass, M. J., & Donner, A. (1994). Evaluation of a palliative care service: Problems and pitfalls. *BMJ*, *309*(6965), 1340–1342.

Magill, L., & Berenson, S. (2008). The conjoint use of music therapy and reflexology with hospitalized advanced stage cancer patients and their families. *Palliative & Supportive Care*, *6*(3), 289–296.

Maue-Johnson, E. L., & Tanguay, C. L. (2006). Assessing the unique needs of hospice patients: A tool for music therapists. *Music Therapy Perspectives*, *24*(1), 13–20.

Monroe, B. (2014). Foreword. In N. Hartley (Ed.), *End of life care: A guide for therapists, artists and arts therapists* (pp. 9–10). Jessica Kingsley Publishers.

Moss, H. (2014). *Aesthetic deprivation: The role of the arts for older people in hospital* [Unpublished doctoral dissertation]. Trinity College Dublin School of Medicine.

Moss, H., Nolan, E., & O'Neill, D. (2007). A cure for the soul? The benefit of live music in the general hospital. *Irish Medical Journal*, *100*(10), 634–636.

Munro, S., & Mount, B. (1978). Music therapy in palliative care. *Canadian Medical Association Journal*, *119*(9), 1029–1034.

Murray, S. A., Kendall, M., Boyd, K., & Sheikh, A. (2005). Illness trajectories and palliative care. *BMJ*, *330*(7498), 1007–1011.

The National Council for Palliative Care. (2015). http://www.ncpc.org.uk/palliative-care-explained

NHS Estates Design Brief Working Group. (2005). *A place to die with dignity: Creating a supportive environment*. NHS Estates.

Nguyen, J. T. (2003). *Effect of music therapy on end-of-life patients' quality of life, emotional state, and family satisfaction as measured by self-report* [Unpublished master's thesis]. Florida State University.

O'Callaghan, C. C. (1996). Lyrical themes in songs written by palliative care patients. *Journal of Music Therapy*, *33*(2), 74–92.

O'Callaghan, C. (2009). Objectivist and constructivist music therapy research in oncology and palliative care: An overview and reflection. *Music and Medicine*, *1*(1), 41–60.

O'Callaghan, C., Forrest, L., & Wen, Y. (2015). Music therapy at the end of life. In B. Wheeler (Ed.), *Music therapy handbook* (pp. 468–480). Guildford Press.

O'Callaghan, C., & Magill, L. (2009). Effect of music therapy on oncologic staff bystanders: A substantive grounded theory. *Palliative & Supportive Care*, *7*(2), 219–228.

O'Callaghan, C., McDermott, F., Hudson, P., & Zalcberg, J. R. (2013). Sound continuing bonds with the deceased: The relevance of music, including preloss music therapy, for eight bereaved caregivers. *Death Studies*, *37*(2), 101–125.

O'Callaghan, C., Petering, H., Thomas, A., & Crappsley, R. (2009). Dealing with palliative care patients' incomplete music therapy legacies: Reflexive group supervision research. *Journal of Palliative Care*, *25*(3), 197–205.

O'Callaghan, C., & Michael, N. (2017). Music therapy in grief and mourning. In J. Edwards (Ed.), *The Oxford handbook of music therapy* (pp. 403–414). Oxford University Press.

O'Kelly, J., & Koffman, J. (2007). Multidisciplinary perspectives of music therapy in adult palliative care. *Palliative Medicine*, *21*(3), 235–241.

Paul, S., & Sallnow, L. (2013). Public health approaches to end-of-life care in the UK: An online survey of palliative care services. *BMJ Supportive & Palliative Care*, *3*(2), 196–199.

Pavlicevic, M., Tsiris, G., Wood, S., Powell, H., Graham, Sanderson, R. J., Millman, R., & Gibson, J. (2015). The 'ripple effect': Towards researching improvisational music therapy in dementia care-homes. *Dementia: The International Journal of Social Research and Practice*, *14*(5), 659–679.

Peng, C. (2018) Our shared humanity—Music as a means of facilitating conversations on end-of-life care. *JAMA Oncology*, *4*(6), 771–772.

Popkin, K., Levin, T., Lichtenthal, W. G., Redl, N., Rothstein, H. D., Siegel, D., & Coyle, N. (2011). A pilot music therapy-centered grief intervention for nurses and ancillary staff working in cancer settings. *Music and Medicine*, *3*(1), 40–46.

Porter, S., McConnell, T., Graham-Wisener, L., Regan, J., McKeown, M., Kirkwood, J., … & Reid, J. (2018). A randomised controlled pilot and feasibility study of music therapy for improving the quality of life of hospice inpatients. *BMC Palliative Care*, *17*(1), 1–9.

Rawlence, C. (2007). John's song. In L. Jarrett (Ed.), *Creative engagement in palliative care: New perspectives on user involvement* (pp. 3–10). Radcliffe.

Salau, S., Rumbold, B., & Young, B. (2007). From concept to care: Enabling community care through a health promoting palliative care approach. *Contemporary Nurse*, *27*(1), 132–140.

Sallnow, L., Kumar, S., & Kellehear, A. (Eds.). (2013). *International perspectives on public health and palliative care*. Routledge.

Saunders, C. (1967). *The management of terminal illness*. Hospital Medicine Publications.

Schmid, W. (2018). Meeting complexity with collaboration: A proposed conceptual framework for participatory community-based music therapy research in end of life-care. *Qualitative Research in Medicine and Healthcare*, *2*(3), 145–153.

Schmid, W., & Ostermann, T. (2010). Home-based music therapy—A systematic overview of settings and conditions for an innovative service in healthcare. *BMC Health Services Research, 10*(1), 291.

Schmid, W., Rosland, J. H., von Hofacker, S., Hunskår, I., & Bruvik, F. (2018). Patient's and health care provider's perspectives on music therapy in palliative care—An integrative review. *BMC Palliative Care, 17*(1), 32.

Schroeder-Sheker, T. (1994). Music for the dying: A personal account of the new field of music-thanatology—History, theories, and clinical narratives. *Journal of Holistic Nursing, 12*(1), 83–99.

Shoemark, H. (2009). Sweet melodies: Combining the talents and knowledge of music therapy and elite musicianship. *Voices: A World Forum for Music Therapy, 9*(2). https://doi.org/10.15845/voices.v9i2.347

Silverman, M. J., & Furman, A. G. (2014). Employment and membership trends in the American Music Therapy Association, 1998–2009. *Music Therapy Perspectives, 32*(1), 99–108.

Simard, J. (2014). *The end-of-life Namaste Care program for people with dementia.* Health Professions Press.

Skånland, M. S. (2012). *A technology of well-being: A qualitative study on the use of MP3 players as a medium for musical self-care.* Lambert Academic Publishing.

Slivka, H. H., & Magill, L. (1986). The conjoint use of social work and music therapy in working with children of cancer patients. *Music Therapy, 6*(1), 30–40.

Spiro, N., & Schober, M. F. (2014). Perspectives on music and communication: An introduction. *Psychology of Music, 42*(6), 771–775.

St Columba's Hospice Care. (2020). Hospice patients and primary school children discuss death and dying through songwriting. https://stcolumbashospice.org.uk/hospice-patients-and-primary-school-children-discuss-death-and-dying-through-songwriting

Stacpoole, M., Hockley, J., Thompsell, A., Simard, J., & Volicer, L. (2015). The Namaste Care programme can reduce behavioural symptoms in care home residents with advanced dementia. *International Journal of Geriatric Psychiatry, 30*(7), 702–709.

Stacpoole, M., Hockley, J., Thompsell, A., Simard, J., & Volicer, L. (2017). Implementing the Namaste Care Program for residents with advanced dementia: Exploring the perceptions of families and staff in UK care homes. *Annals of Palliative Medicine, 6*(4), 327–339.

Stember, M. (1991). Advancing the social sciences through the interdisciplinary enterprise. *The Social Science Journal, 28*(1), 1–14.

Stige, B. (2005). Participatory action research. In B. Wheeler (Ed.), *Music therapy research* (2nd ed., pp. 404–415). Barcelona Publishers.

Stige, B., Ansdell, G., Elefant, C., & Pavlicevic, M. (2010). *Where music helps: Community music therapy in action and reflection.* Ashgate.

Stjernswärd, J. (2007). Palliative care: The public health strategy. *Journal of Public Health Policy, 28*(1), 42–55.

Tapson, C., Noble, D., Daykin, N., & Walters, D. (2018). *Live Music in Care: The impact of music interventions for people living and working in care home settings.* www.livemusicincare.org.uk

Tsiris, G. (2018). *Performing spirituality in music therapy: Towards action, context and the everyday* [Doctoral dissertation, Nordoff Robbins/Goldsmith's, University of London]. Research Online. http://research.gold.ac.uk/23037

Tsiris, G., Tasker, M., Lawson, V., Prince, G., Dives, T., Sands, M., & Ridley, A. (2011). Music and arts in health promotion and death education: The St Christopher's schools project. *Music and Arts in Action, 3*(2), 95–119.

Tsiris, G., Dives, T., & Prince, G. (2014). Music therapy: Evaluation of staff perceptions at St Christopher's Hospice. *European Journal of Palliative Care, 21*(2), 72–75.

Tsiris, G., & Hartley, N. (2014). Research and evaluation. In N. Hartley (Ed.), *End of life care: A guide for therapists, artists and arts therapists* (pp. 227–254). Jessica Kingsley Publishers.

Tsiris, G., Derrington, P., Sparkes, P., Spiro, N., & Wilson, G. (2016). Interdisciplinary dialogues in music, health and wellbeing: Difficulties, challenges and pitfalls. In M. Belgrave (Ed.), *Proceedings of the ISME Commission on Special Music Education and Music Therapy (20–23 July 2016, Edinburgh, Scotland)* (pp. 58–70). International Society for Music Education.

Tsiris, G., Hastings, D., Chaddock, B., Fischbacher, S., & McLarty, M. (September 18, 2019, 2019). Songwriting for grief and loss: An intergenerational project between hospice patients and primary school children [Poster presentation]. The Scottish Partnership for Palliative Care Conference: Provocation, innovation and eternal truths, Edinburgh, United Kingdom.

Tsiris, G., Spiro, N., Coggins, O., & Zubala, A. (2020). The Impact Areas Questionnaire (IAQ): A music therapy service evaluation tool. *Voices: A World Forum for Music Therapy, 20*(2). https://doi.org10.15845/voices.v20i2.2816

Vist, T., & Bonde, L. O. (2013). 'Then certain songs came': Music listening in the grieving process after losing a child. In L. O. Bonde, E. Ruud, M. S. Skånland, & G. Trondalen (Eds.), *Music life stories: Narratives on health musicking* (pp. 139–163). Norwegian Academy of Music.

Waller, S., & Finn, H. (2011). *Improving the patient experience: Environments for care at end of life*. The King's Fund.

Wigram, T., & Gold, C. (2012). The religion of evidence-based practice: Helpful or harmful to health and wellbeing? In R. MacDonald, G. Kreutz, & L. Mitchell (Eds.), *Music, health, and wellbeing* (pp. 164–182). Oxford University Press.

Wlodarczyk, N. (2007). The effect of music therapy on the spirituality of persons in an in-patient hospice unit as measured by self-report. *Journal of Music Therapy, 44*(2), 113–122.

Wood, S. (2015). *The performance of community music therapy evaluation* [Unpublished doctoral dissertation]. Nordoff Robbins/City, University of London.

7
Synthesis

The future of musical care

Neta Spiro, Katie Rose M. Sanfilippo, and Ian Cross

This book exemplifies the spectra of who engages in musical care, of the roles musical care can have, and of the activities that can be part of musical care. It presents examples of musical care throughout the life course with people with a vast range of lived experience; from premature babies in the neonatal intensive care unit (NICU), to children attending school, to adolescents with mental health issues, to adults taking care of their own well-being, to older adults with breathing issues, and to the familial considerations of those at the end of their lives. Thus, this book suggests the potential relevance of musical care to everyone.

With this richness in mind, we begin with discussion of the ebb and flow of the place of musical care throughout the life course. We bring together the ideas presented throughout the book in terms of outcome, context, focus of care, and musical activities. We then go on to introduce two models of disciplinary relationships within musical care, and develop further the conceptualization of musical care. Then comes consideration of the book's limitations, which leads to identification of opportunities. These opportunities include implications of the term musical care; the use of the life stage structure; to whom musical care is relevant, and where, when, and why; and the importance of considering cultural context for future work. We close by bringing together suggestions for future work with a final call to action.

Musical care throughout the life course

The chapters highlight the evolving place—the ebb and flow of outcomes, scope, musical activities, and contexts—of musical care throughout the life course. Issues of cognition, emotion, mental and physical health, identity, education, and relationships receive different levels of attention throughout the book. Issues of development in areas of cognition, emotion, or physical health dominate in life stages in which these are most likely to be developing (e.g., childhood) or challenged (e.g., older adulthood and end of life). Mental health is present throughout the chapters, showing its importance in musical care research and practice throughout the life course. Issues of identity dominate more in adolescence and end of life. Similarly, musical care as self-care

Neta Spiro, Katie Rose M. Sanfilippo, and Ian Cross, *Synthesis* In: *Collaborative Insights*. Edited by: Neta Spiro and Katie Rose M. Sanfilippo, Oxford University Press. © Oxford University Press 2022. DOI: 10.1093/oso/9780197535011.003.0008 is centrally discussed in adulthood but it is also discussed in the context of adolescence as well as those of older adulthood and end of life. This is not to say that areas disappear from other life stages entirely, but merely that, at least in this book, priority is given during certain periods.

Although in some cases the chapters acknowledge the social context (such as other children in school, peers in adolescence, and community members in a care home), most of the chapters focus on care of individuals. In general terms, the focus of care seems to follow an hourglass pattern. The first and final chapters explicitly bring a broader range of people into focus of care. In infancy, caregivers, and especially mothers, are included in considerations of both those who give and receive care. At end of life, the focus of those touched by musical care extends to family members, care staff, and educators, as well as people in the broader environment surrounding end-of-life care. The focus of care thus narrows and widens across the life course—it can specifically attend to individuals or see individuals as part of familial or community groups. More broadly, work considered in some of the life stages—particularly older adulthood and end of life—lends itself to more explicit consideration of the broader influence of musical care, such as musical care touching on carers and other staff in a care home, and acting as consequence of the core care activities.

All the chapters involve discussion of a wide range of music and music activities. Activities range from the more informal, everyday uses of music, such as private or group music listening, to the more formal, such putting on concerts in care homes. They range from the more public, such as singing in community choirs, to the more private, such as caregivers singing with their infants. They also range from the more explicitly therapeutic, such as one-to-one music therapy sessions, to the educational, such as instrumental lessons. Though often studied separately, the more formal, targeted musical care practices grow from the more informal, everyday ones. Indeed, although all these forms of musical care bring their individual practices, expectations, goals, and outcomes, seeing them together highlights the interrelated nature of musical care throughout the life course.

From multi- to interdisciplinary collaboration

Just as we see a multiplicity and ebb and flow of music practices, people, and contexts relevant to musical care, we see a vast range of disciplines that inform the practice and research of musical care. As discussed in the Introduction, collaborations occur across a spectrum from multi- to transdisciplinary work (Choi and Pak, 2006; Rosenfield, 1992). Different types of collaborations bring with them different degrees of communication and sharing, as well as different degrees of cooperation and interaction. We would expect collaboration to be easier in areas that already have teams that have experience of communication and cooperation across disciplines (Aboelela et al., 2007). In some contexts, because of the situation or life stage, we see a drawing together of disciplines; the person receiving musical care attracts a range of disciplines that act together in what we call the *magnet model* of disciplinary relationships. In other contexts, several disciplines can be relevant to musical care or its research and are likely to run alongside one another, but are less likely to interact directly. We call this the *concurrent model*.

In infancy, older adulthood, and end of life, we see a dominance of the *magnet model*, with multidisciplinary teams coalescing around individuals in receipt of care. In these cases, we see several disciplines brought into the same research projects. In childhood, we see a dominance of the *concurrent model*, wherein several fields—child psychology, education, and social development—are present but less often coalesce in the same research projects. Of course, neither the *magnet model* nor the *concurrent model* accounts for all examples of research in a given life stage. For example, in childhood, children in special schools are likely to have a multidisciplinary team coalescing around them, representing an example of the *magnet model*. Nevertheless, from the research drawn on throughout the book, it seems to us that interdisciplinary research may so far have been more common and perhaps easier if the disciplinarily relationships follow a *magnet model* rather than a *concurrent model*.

Just as the relationships between disciplines vary, so do the disciplines themselves. We see disciplines related directly to practice (e.g., mental health, paediatrics, obstetrics and gynaecology, nursing, and education). We also see research from the academic worlds of music research (e.g., music psychology, music sociology, and ethnomusicology), and from broader academic research (e.g., psychology, neuroscience, and sociology). Some contexts and life stages attract more emphasis on multidisciplinary collaboration with non-music-practice-led fields while others have greater focus on the academic, be it more general or music specific. For example, in NICU work in infancy, paediatrics, obstetrics and gynaecology, and mental health are all present in care and are part of multidisciplinary research in the area. Similarly, in institutional end-of-life care, nursing and palliative care are integral to the practice and theory of musical care. In contrast, examples from everyday uses of music in adolescence can happen quite independently of other practices and much research draws on academic work such as music psychology. Similarly, in adulthood, examples of musical self-care draw on academic research in sociology. This is not to say that these broad research areas are relevant only in certain contexts. For example, non-musical, practice-led research fields are relevant in adolescence (talking therapies and occupational therapies are drawn on). Similarly, other academic fields are present in infancy (e.g., music psychology, developmental psychology). But the chapters of this book illustrate the breadth of disciplines relevant to musical care, and it is striking, given the broad range of relevant fields, how little explicit interdisciplinary collaboration is reported, be it with non-music-practice-led or academically based disciplines.

Perhaps, though, it is not surprising that there is little explicit interdisciplinary collaboration. If nothing else, there are several challenges that can stand in the way (see, for example, MacLeod, 2018; Powell et al., 1999). One challenge is connected to the interpretation of terms. As a basic example, what is referred to when we consider 'music' can vary widely; from a focus on the sounds heard to an understanding involving all bodily movements and expression. Technical terms in the field—from the broadest to the most specific—can have numerous formal definitions and informal associations. Consider, for example, interpretations of the terms emotion, communication, interaction, mechanisms, entrainment, and dissonance. Using the same terms with overlapping but not identical meanings can lead to researchers thinking they share conceptual assumptions, when in fact key issues distinguish their thinking. Similarly, with mismatches in use of terms, researchers can think that they fundamentally disagree with one another, when in fact they are closer in their understanding (Spiro and Schober, 2014; Tsiris et al., 2016): one person's mechanism may be another's process; one person's significant difference is another's striking change.

A further difficulty can be in the understanding of the purpose of the research (for example, King et al., 2008; Nyström et al., 2018). For some, more often the practice-led work, a key focus is on understanding musical care in particular cases and situations; how can the research contribute to understanding and improving care for this person or this situation? For others, more often the more theory-led work, the questions are broader, focusing on how the research can contribute to our general understanding of musical care—how and why it might occur—and on generalizable claims, or claims that go beyond individuals.

Connected to the difficulties in the different priorities of research are questions about what can be taken as the basis for trustworthy conclusions (as discussed in Bindler et al., 2012; Petticrew and Roberts, 2003). Each research project involves choices about methodological approaches (Hesse-Biber, 2016). These include choices about whose views are important and at what stage of a project those perspectives are incorporated. The choices are also about what kinds of measures are relevant and respected. Further choices concern where and how information is collected, as well as where and how the research is shared and for what purpose. Researchers' views may differ about each of these key points. For example, for some researchers, the claim that music contributes to care in particular ways requires the systematic comparison of outcome (often by using numeric, validated measures) of matched participant groups that have experienced a music activity with those that have not, as seen in randomized controlled trials. For others, the claim that music helps in particular ways requires getting to know all of those involved in the process through, for example, ethnographic approaches of immersing oneself in particular settings and/or carrying out interviews. For some, the presentation of clear hypotheses that can be tested with a predetermined, publicly registered protocol is the way to test theories about the impact of musical care. For others the process of learning about an intervention as it happens, using grounded theory work from which the questions themselves emerge from the data is the way to understand the process and impact of musical care.

These issues of trustworthiness of findings are not limited to explicitly interdisciplinary work. As in other areas of research, there are plenty of areas of controversy in the realm of music and its effects (see, for example, the debates that followed the publication of a paper, 'Music and Spatial Task Performance'; Rauscher et al., 1993, or Cochrane reviews such as Magee et al., 2017 that question the quality of evidence and suggest that more research is needed before recommendations for clinical practice can be made).

With this broad view of musical care, we see that music *can* play a role in a vast range of settings. Or to put it another way, many of the studies in the field illustrate that music *can* play a role in particular contexts—not that it necessarily always does in every context for everyone. It may be that other art forms or other activities are more relevant in particular instances. Indeed, identifying the limits of where music can help does not negate the role of music in general. This broad view of musical care perhaps invites a variegated view of music—identifying where it does or does not play particular roles. Indeed, in many of the forms of engagement discussed in the book, the primary reason for engagement is not just (or even at all) for care reasons. In terms of applicable advice, this point seems important. It also seems to us that there are several reasons to carry out research in this field: it has potential to lead to practical implications for formal musical care work and to provide advice for informal musical engagement. It also has a more fundamental purpose: helping us understand what happens when we engage in music and thus understanding why we may have it and value it.

Projects can use one or a number of methods, whether they are single-, multi- or interdisciplinary. Interdisciplinary work involves explicitly going beyond the methodological choices to take in the exchange and integration of knowledge from the start of a project, whether it be about research approaches, theories, assumptions, or priorities (Choi and Pak, 2006; Rosenfield, 1992). All of the disciplines drawn on in this book have a variegated field of researchers with their own priorities, proclivities, and values.

Taken together, these areas of difference, and sometimes strong disagreement, can be seen as connected to underlying perspectives, ideologies, and beliefs about musical care, research, and practice. These broad views can then influence specific choices about terms, methods, and approaches. For example, the term intervention can be seen as a broad category to describe any activity that is thought to (usually positively) affect the outcome or course of a condition or process. For others, it is a term that fits within the biomedical model of health and brings with it assumptions associated with that model. As exemplified in this book, the area of musical care includes within it a range of attitudes to this term and all that comes with it. These ideologically informed differences are not unique to musical care and can even be seen from within the same areas of expertise. For example, in the nearby area of expert music performance, in a case study in which players had just improvised on a jazz standard, they held quite different views about the description and assignment of intentions, about who has responsibility for what happens, and about how much is 'predetermined', ideas that seemed ideologically informed (Schober and Spiro, 2014).

These areas of commonalities and tensions exemplify both the challenges and opportunities of interdisciplinary dialogue and work in the communities surrounding musical care. On an individual level, it is possible for researchers from different disciplines to find themselves more closely aligned with one another than with others in their individual disciplines (Spiro and Schober, 2014). Indeed, as the chapters in this book illustrate, the overlaps in understanding that can occur among researchers and practitioners from different disciplines can be so substantial that the boundaries usually drawn around the individual disciplines fade away. Interdisciplinary research can bridge the differences in terminology, focus of work, methodological approaches, and perhaps even ideological perspectives. Therefore, interdisciplinary work, not-withstanding its challenges, seems particularly suited to addressing the multiplicity of questions of the multifaced phenomenon of musical care.

From blurred to broken boundaries

This book began with the invitation to consider the blurred boundaries between different areas of musical care. Seeing the work that the chapters brought together encourages a more radical view. To fully understand musical care, it is helpful to re-move the boundaries altogether. We can see musical care as a whole. Music therapy, music in education, community music, music in health, and musical engagement in daily life can be seen as different parts of a whole, not just as individual and some-times overlapping areas of practice.

More radically still, it is our contention that musical care can be seen as part of a broader whole: part of the spectrum of music making, not a type of musical engage-ment that is separate from other music-making. This view can fundamentally alter the place of musical care. This is not necessarily a niche, separable part of music ac-tivity. In this view, the very notions and definitions of what music is and its place(s) in our culture are reconsidered and broadened. In turn, as discussed further in the next section, these ideas invite a broader range of research questions and consideration of practice in musical care.

Similarly, questions that have so far been limited to music made in musical care contexts become relevant to other music, too. For example, as we have seen here, the role and importance of musical care shifts throughout the life course. How does all this extend to understanding the (shifting) roles of music in our lives more generally? Studying musical care contexts can raise issues and propose theories and potential frameworks that are relevant beyond those contexts. For example, work that begins in musical care contexts—such as looking at interaction in music therapy—can lead to the development of frameworks that may well be applicable in a broader range of contexts of the study of social interaction (e.g., Spiro and Himberg, 2016).

Seeing music in this way is not to propose that we collapse all music engagement into an undifferentiated mess; from some perspectives the distinctions are very important. Rather, it is to propose seeing the different activities as part of a whole. Bringing out what is shared may also highlight with more clarity the idiosyncrasies of musics and of different peoples' engagements in music in different contexts. This broadening out may also shape choices about what kinds of music practices are seen as worthy of attention, study, and support.

From limitations to opportunities

Musical care

In this book, we introduced the term musical care and defined it as the role of music—music listening as well as music-making—in supporting any aspect of people's developmental or health needs. When we use the term musical care, we have to consider what we mean by 'music'. Although all known societies engage in activities that, from a Western perspective, appear to be musical, the musics of different cultures can take very different forms and may appear to fulfil very different functions. Each society seems to have quite specific expectations and beliefs about, and functional roles for, the phenomena that we might term 'music' (see, for example, Nettl 2015).

Although the term musical care is intended to break down boundaries between different practices and contexts, it is limited in its underlying assumption: it is focusing on a positive side of musical engagement. We are heartened, however, that even with this focus implied, Saarkillio and McFerran in their chapter Musical care in adolescence highlight the potential unhelpful uses of music. Similarly, Wood and Clift, in their chapter Musical care in older adulthood, acknowledge that there are limitations to what musical care can do.

Is the introduction of a new term really necessary? As we see it, a new term may be inevitable in a quest for interdisciplinary perspectives on the field. Existing terms are either too specific—music therapy, music in health, community music—or too broad—music. From some perspectives, research on specific music practices is highly pressured—with an eye to funding, evidence gathering, or proving the worth of work. The new term reflects the notion that we are not looking at a boundaried set of activities, practices, or professions, or work that is relevant only to people with diagnoses, in particular situations, or to particular types of music. By using the term musical care, we are looking at overlapping areas of practice and engagement that are widely applicable. And in so doing, as we have seen illustrated in the chapters of this book, we can take a nuanced view on musical care—incorporating its uncertainties, limitations, and problems along with possibilities.

Life course

In this book we used the life stage structure. Taking this view has the danger of encompassing more than any individual chapter can cover in a book of this length. In a book like this one, it is not possible to fully account for every aspect of musical care for each life stage and so choices have been made as to what to prioritize. For an obvious example, we have not heard about the full range of clinical examples of musical care in each life stage. Furthermore, we made choices about which life stages to segment the life course into—we could have used more or fewer, as discussed in the Introduction.

Additionally, of course, while the first five chapters are associated with age ranges, the final—end of life—can occur at any moment.

While the book uses the life stage structure, musical care can in fact be cross-generational. Mothers, parents, and caregivers are considered in the chapter Musical care in infancy, and children and grandchildren are considered in the chapter Musical care at the end of life. So, our boundaries of life stage are as ripe for breaking as those of musical practice, context, and situation.

Beyond the general ebbs and flows of themes mentioned earlier in this synthesis, there are common theories applicable across the life stages. For example, references to communication appear in almost every chapter. The references come from several perspectives, but the same theories come up more than once. For example, the same theories about music's communicative affordances within care interactions are drawn on. Specifically, 'communicative musicality' (Malloch and Trevarthen, 2009) is explicitly referred to in almost every chapter. Indeed, beyond this book, communicative musicality has been applied in several life stages (Trevarthen and Malloch, 2000). In parallel, communicative skills that can be developed through musical care are explored in chapters such as Musical care in childhood and Musical care in adolescence. At the same time, the use of music to communicate messages is also explored, such as in education about maternal mental and physical health in the chapter Musical care in infancy and about death and dying in the chapter Musical care at the end of life.

Ideas and tools presented in this book in the context of only one life stage may also be applicable in other life stages. For example, the Healthy Unhealthy Music Scale (HUMS; Saarikallio et al., 2015) was originally developed for adolescence and is here described solely in that context. The scale, however, has also been used with adults and a different view on musical care would likely have highlighted the similarities and differences of the results of using the scale at these different life stages (Silverman, 2020).

Equally, by taking the life course view, changes in concepts and their application can be brought out. For example, though sharing core characteristics, communication in parent-infant interaction is different from that among adolescents, which is different again from that among carers and older people living with dementia. These differences speak to how music is experienced and used differently throughout the life course. Other examples of such variability include the changes in how musical reward can be experienced (Belfi et al., 2021) and how our preference for, quality judgements of, and emotional reactions to music can change throughout our lives (Krumhansl and Zupnick, 2013). Despite the limitations of the life course structure used in this book, these connections still emerge as reflecting the fact that discrete temporal categories are interconnected. This juxtaposition thus highlights examples of areas of similarity across the life course; the roles that perhaps different types of music engagement can play in, for example, social bonding (Savage et al., 2020) and well-being (Malloch and Trevarthen, 2009; Trevarthen and Malloch, 2000) throughout our lives.

The life course structure has not been systemically used in discussion of research and practices in the broad arena of musical care before. We prioritize the experiences within the life stages over the diagnoses and contexts usually associated with them, thus starting with a more holistic view. As discussed in the Introduction of this book, this view provides the opportunity to highlight the transformations and changes in musical care as life progresses.

Practitioners in and around musical care

The music practice authors in this book are mainly music therapists. Of course, the world of musical care is much broader both in terms of background of musicians (including, for example, community musicians) and in the professionals and others engaging in musical care (be they nurses, family members, or individuals for their own care). Though the chapters provide broad overviews of musical care at each life stage, the perspectives of the authors here are rather similar—indeed, several trained at Nordoff Robbins Music Therapy in London, United Kingdom. It is striking to us that even with this similar background, which perhaps acts as one of the aspects that contributes to coherence in the book, the variety of research and practices presented is broad. In fact, different types of content, research approach, and even writing styles are illustrated throughout the book. The Musical care in infancy and Musical care in adulthood chapters, for example, are quite different in the kinds of topics they choose to focus on, the research fields they draw on, the type of perspective they take, and the style of writing.

Similarly, the range of non-music-led disciplines amongst our authors is small. Most are academics in music psychology, public health, education, or sociology, with one nurse. Almost all of the authors writing together here knew one another, or of one another's work, before they wrote these chapters—a pragmatic choice, given the challenges of true interdisciplinary working. Our hope is that this book will lead to the exploration of further collaborative opportunities—perhaps across disciplines that are further apart. As the field of research develops, we envisage other voices coming through more regularly as co-authors—participants, clients, family members, policy-makers. Thus, the range of collaborators across disciplines will only increase.

Cultural diversity

We invited authors to write chapters in this book who are currently working in only five countries, three of which are primarily English speaking—Australia, Finland, Israel, the United Kingdom, and the United States. This book is not unusual in its focus and follows a long research tradition of restriction to a particular subset of experiences (Henrich et al., 2010). The brief to authors was to give an overview of research in the field, with a focus on interdisciplinary perspectives, and was not to provide a systematic review. The individual chapters vary in the extent to which they bring in examples of, or mention, non-Western musical care practices or seldom-heard communities. While a primary focus on Western care practices contributes to a sense of coherence in the book, and places some kind of temporary boundary in an area that we have already so broadened, many important pieces of what musical care can look, feel, and sound like are missing in this account. That is not to say that the communities represented in this book are homogenous. Indeed, by definition, much research in the area of musical care has in its orbit a wider range of people and musics than other areas of the study of music.

Most work on musical care tends to be conducted from a contemporary Western cultural perspective. However, a significant exception is musical care in infancy, for which research and practice have drawn on experiences from several cultures. As a result, as noted in the Musical care in infancy chapter, there is acknowledgement that the practices of natural musical care that frame interactions between caregivers and infants seem to show similarities across a range of cultures. This acknowledgement stands as something of an exception in the literature of musical care in non-Western societies, in which, generally, explorations of the use of music in caring situations have tended to focus on individual and culture-specific sets of practices (see, e.g., Bahr and Haefer, 1978; Sandlana, 2014; Walker, 2003).

A cross-cultural perspective, in our view, is fundamentally important for a comprehensive understanding of musical care throughout the life course. Therefore, in the following sections we discuss frameworks for understanding musical care across cultures, present a biocultural perspective on musical care throughout the human life course, and explore cross-cultural perspectives on forms of music engagement in musical care.

Musical care across cultures

There have been some attempts to identify possible frameworks for understanding musical care across cultures. For example, Roseman (2011) seeks to develop a cross-culturally applicable scheme for understanding the ways in which cultural models of dealing with illness, and of using music in pursuit of this, are embedded in everyday practices. In this scheme, an understanding of musical healing that can be applied beyond the boundaries of Western therapeutic practice requires consideration of four axes: the musical, the sociocultural, the performative, and the biomedical. For her, the musical embraces not only cultural practice but also the materiality of music as sound and the human response to sound; the sociocultural reflects the embeddedness of music and its significances in specific cultural contexts, experiences, and traditions; the performative reflects the enacted and interactive nature of music as performance; and the biomedical reflects the processes held to underlie the ameliorative change that is effected through music, which may or may not map straightforwardly onto Western conceptions of the biomedical. Though a focus on music as sound rather than sound, concept, and behaviour (cf. Merriam, 1964) undermines the generalizability of Roseman's framework, it should allow fruitful development of the understanding of music's potential for care in clinical and non-clinical contexts in different societies.

Although music and the ways in which it is used in care exhibit huge diversity across world societies, we might expect commonalities to occur at a range of levels. Humans are, after all, one recently emerged species (Stringer, 2016); we possess common biological endowments and capacities that can be expected to constrain certain aspects of human lifeways irrespective of culture. There are at least three features of our species that we can expect to affect how music might be used in care. First, although human cultures exhibit huge variation, part of the biological heritage of all humans is a capacity for culture, a capacity for social learning (Foley and Mirazón Lahr, 2011; Tomasello, 1999); second, another element of that heritage is a motivation to engage cooperatively with others (Tomasello and Vaish, 2013); and finally, perhaps the most evident feature is the common trajectory of the biological changes that occur across our life course. In our use of the term musical care, we encompass the different ways music is used for care across cultures. Though they are not the explicit focus of the chapters of the book, here we highlight some commonalities and differences in the ways in which musical care might be applicable across cultures as well as the life course, thus highlighting opportunities for future work in this area.

A biocultural perspective on musical care throughout the life course

Humans are secondarily altricial (Dunsworth, et al. 2012; Gould, 1983); we are born quite unable to fend for ourselves and with a great deal of growing to do, yet with capacities to sense, and to interact with, caregivers and our auditory environments from birth (see, e.g., Malloch and Trevarthen, 2009; Mampe, et al. 2009). Human infants have profound needs for early care, and an urgent need and capacity to be assimilated into the societies into which they are born, learning culture-appropriate modes of cognition, communication, and interaction. Music can be seen to play significant roles in both early care (as noted in the Musical care in infancy chapter) and in processes of childhood socialization across cultures; linguistic and musical modes of interaction are most likely indistinguishable in early life stages (Brandt et al., 2012), and those few studies that have explored the ways in which music or its emic equivalent function for young children in non-Western societies have shown it to be central to their socialization. In two very different African societies—the agrarian Venda (Blacking, 1967) and the hunter-gatherer Mbendjele (Lewis, 2009), musical activities were found both to bring young people together and to enable them to prepare for and rehearse aspects of their adult social selves.

These two particular societies might be seen as particularly cooperative and involving high levels of mutual dependency between culture members; other societies may place more value on self-determination and freedom of choice, and music, and musical care, may take other forms and serve other functions, or even be valued differently. The idea that cultures may be characterized by the extent to which their members exhibit individualistic or collectivist traits was proposed by Triandis et al. (1988) to account for cultures' internal structures and dynamics. As Kitayama and Marcus (2010) note, selves both constitute and are constituted by their environments and particularly their cultural environments. From that perspective, it would be unsurprising if music were to be found to play different caring roles in cultures that tended more towards the collectivist than the individualistic, and vice versa. On the other hand, the large-scale study of Vignoles et al. (2016, p. 967) showed that 'a simple contrast between independence and interdependence does not adequately capture the diverse models of selfhood that prevail in different world regions'. They suggest that a more fine-grained approach enables more accurate predictions about, for example, how well-being in a given culture may be linked more closely either to general self-efficacy or to the privileging of harmonious relationships. The prevalence within particular societies of these types of difference in construal of well-being could thus implicate different ways of engaging with music as being more, or less, efficacious in care contexts according to the self-constituting dynamics of different societies.

Notwithstanding whether or not a particular society tends towards individualism, collectivism, or some more complex construct, it appears that all humans are subject to a quite specific social need: the need to belong (Baumeister and Leary, 1995). Humans appear to require a sense of connectedness to others to underpin their own sense of well-being, and it's thus likely that music will be capable of motivating that sense of belonging irrespective of broader societal dynamics. Music, particularly in the participatory form (Turino, 2008) that involves making music together, seems to elicit a sense of social bonding between participants, and an increasing number of studies are confirming that finding in children (as discussed in the Musical care in childhood chapter, and in Rabinowitch et al., 2013) and in adults (e.g., Hove and Risen, 2009; Schäfer and Eerola, 2018). In effect, it appears that across cultures music constitutes an excellent means of managing situations of social uncertainty (Cross, 2006) by bringing about or enhancing a sense of social solidarity between culture members. It's likely that, however much the differences in the specific dynamics of cultures lead to differences in conceptions of well-being and care, music's capacity to manage situations of social uncertainty still endows it with a broad efficacy in caring processes that acknowledge the social dimension.

Our infant and childhood patterns of dependency on others to meet our needs (including those for care) can be grounded securely in our uniquely human biologies. Rather more surprisingly, a further life stage, adolescence, appears to be unique to humans. Bogin (1994, 1999) suggests that this particular life stage (typified by its species-specific growth spurt) arose as an evolutionary adaption to accommodate the substantial amount of social and cultural learning necessary to deal with the complexities of adult human social life. Though foundationally biological, adolescence is unambiguously a cultural construction, as Lesko, (2012) notes. Its implications, as a matrix of agentive identity formation during a life stage of radical biological change, appear to vary radically in the contexts of different cultures and it can be expected that this variability will bear significantly on the ways in which adolescents relate to, and relate to one another through, music in different cultural contexts. Indeed, Boer et al. (2012) found that amongst adolescents from six quite diverse cultural samples (Germany, Kenya, Mexico, New Zealand, Philippines, and Turkey), there was limited variation across cultures in the ways in which music served social functions for young people (such as development of individual values, or for bonding with peers), but significant variability according to country in the ways in which music fulfilled sociocultural functions (such as marking cultural identity, or effecting family bonding). A subsequent cross-cultural study of music listening by adolescents in family and peer groups (Boer and Abubakar, 2014) found that music listening in both contexts contributed to cohesion in their respective groups. However, music listening in peer groups contributed to well-being across cultural contexts, whereas musical family rituals affect emotional well-being primarily in more traditional or collectivistic contexts.

It has to be noted that such effects are likely to be susceptible to change in the light of the increasing globalization of remote and private access to music (and music video) afforded by the increasing ubiquity of connectedness to the Internet. Even since 2000 there have been radical changes in the ways in which we can access and engage with music and engage with others through music. These factors are likely to have significant impacts on the ways in which music can be used (particularly for self-care) by adolescents (as discussed in the Musical care in adolescence chapter), impacts that are only now beginning to be explored. For example, Harris and Cross (2021), using a paradigm in which participants collaborated with a fictive partner in making playlists, showed that the belief that they were interacting with another human being could enhance participants' sense of connectedness to their supposed collaborator but that this effect seemed to be limited to younger participants for whom remote playlist-making had simply become part of their cultural landscape. Although we might anticipate similar age-dependent effects of technological change on the efficacy of musical care that is more or less independent of culture, we need to maintain an awareness of the extent to which music accessibility and disseminability is mediated by commercial considerations and may involve unacknowledged and potentially damaging transactions (see, e.g., Drott, 2018; Fleischer, 2017) that co-opt and undermine adolescent autonomy in engaging with music.

Across cultures, activities that appear to us to be musical take a wide range of forms and fulfil diverse functions that help centre self, and equilibrate social norms with sense of self, facilitating well-being. The emergence of individual identity as an autonomous social self, partially shaped by music, is likely to provide the roots for the flourishing of that autonomous social self in adulthood (as discussed in the Musical care in adulthood chapter), though the nature of the individual engagement with music will vary widely from culture to culture and from one social context to another.

Cross-cultural perspectives on forms of music engagement in musical care

Turino (2008) introduced a very useful distinction between presentational and participatory musics; the former involves a clear distinction between performers and audience, while the latter allows for community-wide participation in music-making with all serving both as performers and audience members. In contemporary Western cultures the 'standard' conception of music tends to be based on music as presentational—music produced by specialists that is listened to or consumed by the general public. Conversely, in traditional or rural societies, participatory forms of music-making are often thought to be much more common. Nevertheless, participatory music is much more prevalent in Western societies than is often thought to be the case (Finnegan, 1989), whereas the global spread of music in recorded and broadcast form has rendered presentational music pretty much ubiquitous; both forms are likely to play significant roles in everyday uses of music across most cultures and, as we have seen in earlier chapters, both forms are commonly used in care contexts.

From the later 19th century, developments in the technology of recording, reproducing, and producing music as sound (Katz, 2010) have led to the predominant mode of engagement with music worldwide becoming presentational, with solitary musical listening becoming widespread. This predominance could be interpreted as an impoverishment of the musical experience in modern times; after all, until the mid-19th century, if you wanted to experience music you either did it yourself or paid someone to produce it for you, but in either case music had the potential to be experienced as live and interactive. From such a perspective, solitary musical listening could be regarded as somewhat pathological. However, in many societies other than those of the contemporary West, solitary listening, or making music solely for oneself ('holicipation', in Killick's [2006] terminology), is a common mode of engagement with music. In societies as widespread as those of the Batek (hunter-gatherers in tropical Malaysia: see Rudge, 2019), or of the Nenets (reindeer-herding nomads in northern arctic Russia: see Abramovich-Gomon, 1999), solitary music-making is prevalent. Indeed, as Abramovitch-Gomon notes (1999, p. 37), even in Nenets' public performance amongst groups of friends and family, 'singers still behave as if they are singing for themselves, deeply immersed in the performance, as if possessed by the characters and events of the stories'. Hence solitary music-making and listening can be regarded as at least as 'natural', and prospectively efficacious in care, as any group participatory form of music.

That being said, it does appear that participatory forms are significant in establishing or reaffirming the social equilibrium. Music-making is a key element in ceremonies and rituals that accompany or consummate life stage transitions in almost every culture, when individuals move from pubescence to adolescence, from single to married states, or from life to death. Participatory music serves, as Nettl (2015, p. 253) puts it, to 'support the integrity of social groups', managing situations of social uncertainty in which potential outcomes may threaten that integrity (Cross, 2006). More mundanely, regular rituals such as those involved in everyday religious observance are likely to involve music as a means of reconstituting the sense of self in relation to the community, again minimizing perceived social uncertainty. Other regular, though secular, rituals, such as following one's team at a football match, may again involve the use of music in the form of football songs or chants (see Clark, 2006; Kytö, 2011) to help establish and project a sense of group identity. All these forms of participatory involvement in music-making can be co-opted in the context of care, and all are evident in most world cultures.

A cross-cultural view of musical care suggests to us paths for potential areas of development in research in musical care throughout the life course and across cultures. Beyond the obvious blind spots, a humbler approach to research in musical care, learning about musical care in a broader range of cultural contexts, can inform our understanding of musical care in Western contexts. If nothing else, questioning assumptions about, for example, how people can interact or how information can be shared may lead to alternative ways of thinking about, and practicing, musical care, and at the very least being more specific about levels of generalizability of claims. Put in more extreme terms, what counts as musical care, and therefore who counts as being relevant for research, needs to be considered. We envisage that these issues of representation will be central concerns of a subsequent volume of *Collaborative Insights*.

We see substantial opportunities in this interdisciplinary, collaborative view; bringing in a broader range of voices and perspectives can enhance our understanding of musical care and bring into focus practices and people that have previously been sidelined. More dramatically still, this broadening of focus has implications not only for our understanding of musical care, but also for music more generally.

From future directions to a call to action

This book is intended not just as a retrospective view of research, but also as a call to action: an invitation to new interdisciplinary research paths. Each chapter therefore leads to an explicit summary of possible future work relevant to each life stage, but taking the chapters together several common themes emerge.

Interdisciplinary research

Not surprisingly, given the focus of the book, all the chapters point out the promise of interdisciplinary research. The chapters illustrate what has been learned from interdisciplinary research, as well as its relative lack in the field. The need for interdisciplinary research was clear in the context of, for example, multidisciplinary work we have characterized as being represented by the *magnet model* of collaboration. As highlighted in the Musical care in infancy chapter, in the NICU in infancy, more explicit interdisciplinary collaboration amongst medical personnel, music therapists, and families is essential for music therapy to become part of standard care in the NICU. Similarly, in the Musical care at the end of life chapter, the authors highlight the importance of the synthesis of approaches to ensure both the maintenance and mutual enriching of multiple practices, theoretical perspectives, and professional frameworks. The approaches here include music-based disciplines and other fields, such as nursing and spiritual care.

Other contexts that call for more interdisciplinary research emerged from what we characterized as the *concurrent model* of collaboration. In such cases, interdisciplinary research can apply theories or practices identified in one discipline to address a gap in another. For example, as discussed in the Musical care in childhood chapter, despite the focus on music and emotion research in music psychology and related fields, the authors identify a gap in the ways in which musical care is understood to play a role in children's social-emotional development. This gap concerns an understanding of the effects of different kinds of music, kinds of musical interactions, and modes of engagement, on children's social-emotional development.

Combining methods

Several chapters point out the potential for incorporation of different methods in, and even specific tools for, research. As pointed out in the Musical care at the end of life chapter, there is potential to diversify methods to include service evaluation and arts-based methods. Doing so would prioritize and promote user involvement by engaging with the people who make the hospice community, including patients, their families, staff, and the local community.

As pointed out in the chapter Musical care in adulthood, ethnographic and ethnomusicological approaches focus on details of music as it occurs in particular social situations. While this methodological approach to musical care research allows focus on how musical care is achieved in practice, how music is understood as a means of care, and the role of mutuality in musical care, as Procter and DeNora point out, this methodological approach needs to be brought together with work that focuses on the effects of musical care.

Studying the effects of musical care is not straightforward. As highlighted in the chapter on Musical care in childhood, many researchers focus on the importance of randomization in the experimental design as far as practically possible within clinical and educational settings. Real-world applicability is also essential, as is acknowledgement of personal proclivities and preferences, so a balance between research rigor and practical applicability is essential. In many studies, the participants themselves often choose whether or not to participate, which could play a role in any observed behavioural outcomes. Disentangling the various possible contributors to outcomes, be they individual or musical, is a fundamental area for future research.

Several authors present the simultaneous priorities that emerge in the field of musical care: the importance of large-scale, outcomes-based, generalizable investigations of the effects of musical care, the need for methods that respect and help understand the flexible, personal, idiosyncratic, and subtle nature of musical care, and the real-world applicability of research. Combining methods may ease the tensions between different approaches, be they tensions between rigorous scientific approaches and applicability in the moment, or tensions between the flexible nature of musical care and understanding commonalities of experience.

Who, what, where, and for how long is the focus?

We've seen in this book the range of who gets attention within musical care research and practice: from individuals, to parents, to family units, to communities. Nevertheless, the scope for development in future is vast. For example, as highlighted by Sanfilippo et al., in Musical care in infancy, for the most part, research on infant musical care has focused mainly on the mother as the agent of care, whereas, in fact, fathers' place in musical care is not to be dismissed. Indeed, in many situations, as highlighted by Procter and DeNora in Musical care in adulthood, and Tsiris et al. in Musical care at the end of life, consideration of a wider circle (a wider familial or community circle) should be considered.

As pointed out earlier in this chapter and by Sanfilippo et al. in Musical care in infancy, we in the West know much more about Western practices than about non-Western ones. The potential in opening our eyes to non-Western practices is significant. Moreover, as Sanfilippo et al. in Musical care in infancy point out, there is much to be learned from musical care that happens more locally to us but is often overlooked—that which takes place in marginalized or seldom-heard communities. Learning about a wider range of musical practices can inform, and help us question, basic assumptions about what musical care can look like, for whom it can be, where it can take place, and why.

We've seen in this book a wide variety of musical activities. However, the variety of musical activities that occur in musical care is wider still (such as co-created musical activities, technologically mediated work, and guided imagery in music). With this broader scope the commonalities and differences in musical care in this diverse area of music engagement can be brought more fully into view.

We've also seen a wide variety of contexts of musical care: from institutions to homes. Some authors nevertheless point out the lack of research in some settings. As Procter and DeNora highlight in Musical care in adulthood, to fully capture the range of musical care throughout the life course, we need to include the full range of where and when musical care occurs—not just observe it where it is pre-planned. In a specific example, Tsiris et al. in Musical care at the end of life highlight the lack of attention on home-based work for end-of-life care.

Musical care is often a longitudinal activity and yet most research in the area is short term (referring often to one event of musical engagement). As Farrant et al. in Musical care in childhood point out, children engage with music throughout their childhood and beyond. Indeed, as this book highlights, there are several questions about musical care that span several life stages, suggesting that longitudinal views may be particularly enlightening in our understanding of the ebb and flow of the roles of musical care in our lives. How do, for example, the roles of musical care change in relation to our identity, to our social relationships, or to our emotion regulation throughout the life course?

Finally, these chapters have brought out the burgeoning fields of health promotion, communication about health, and community engagement. These came out particularly in the chapters Musical in infancy and Musical care at the end of life, but these fields seem relevant at other stages in the life course as well.

Getting, in our view, to the heart of what we define as musical care, several future directions are about the expansion of who is considered, what musics are included, what contexts are seen as relevant, and which theoretical and methodological approaches are seen as helpful.

A call to action

We end here with the same call to action we began with in the Introduction. Whether you are a practitioner interested in musical care, a music psychologist interested in musical care practice and approaches, a music therapist interested in wider research areas, or a student embarking in any discipline represented in this text, we hope that you feel inspired to engage further with interdisciplinary work and perspectives on musical care. We hope this book will be a catalyst for new collaborations that will bring new insights to musical care throughout the life course.

References

Aboelela, S. W., Larson, E., Bakken, S., Carrasquillo, O., Formicola, A., Glied, S. A., Haas, J., & Gebbe, M. (2007). Defining interdisciplinary research: Conclusions from a critical review of the literature. *Health Services Research, 42*(1), 329–346. https://doi.org/10.1111/j.1475-6773.2006.00621.x

Abramovich-Gomon, A. (1999). *The Nenets' song: A microcosm of a vanishing culture*. Ashgate Publishing.

Bahr, D., & Haefer, J. (1978). Song in Piman curing. *Ethnomusicology, 22*, 89–122.

Baumeister, R., & Leary, M. (1995) The need to belong: Desire for interpersonal attachments as a fundamental human motivation. *Psychological Bulletin, 117*, 497–529.

Belfi, A. M., Moreno, G. L., Gugliano, M., & Neill, C. (2021). Musical reward across the lifespan. *Aging & Mental Health*, 1–8. https://doi.org/10.1080/13607863.2021.1871881

Bindler, R. C., Richardson, B., Daratha, K., & Wordell, D. (2012). Interdisciplinary health science research collaboration: Strengths, challenges, and case example. *Applied Nursing Research, 25*, 95–100. https://doi.org/10.1016/j.apnr.2010.06.004

Blacking, J. (1967). *Venda children's songs: A study in ethnomusicological analysis*. Witwatersrand University Press.

Boer, D., & Abubakar, A. (2014). Music listening in families and peer groups: Benefits for young people's social cohesion and emotional well-being across four cultures. *Frontiers in Psychology, 5*, 392. https://doi.org/10.3389/fpsyg.2014.00392

Boer, D., Fischer, R., Tekman, H. G., Abubaker, A., Nienga, J., & Zenger, M. (2012). Young people's topography of musical functions: Personal, social and cultural experiences with music across genders and six societies. *International Journal of Psychology, 47*(5), 355–369. https://doi.org/10.1080/00207594.2012.656128

Bogin, B. (1994). Adolescence in evolutionary perspective. *Acta Pædiatrica*, *83*, 29–35. https://doi.org/10.1111/j.1651-2227.1994.tb13418.x

Bogin, B. (1999). *Patterns of human growth* (2nd ed.). Cambridge University Press.

Brandt, A., Gebrian, M., & Slevc, L. R. (2012). Music and early language acquisition. *Frontiers in Psychology*, *3*, 1–17. https://doi.org/10.3389/fpsyg.2012.00327

Choi, B. C., & Pak, A. W. (2006). Multidisciplinarity, interdisciplinarity and/transdisciplinarity in health research, services, education and policy: 1. Definitions, objectives, and evidence of effectiveness. *Clinical and Investigative Medicine*, *29*, 351–364.

Clark, T. (2006). 'I'm Scunthorpe 'til I die': Constructing and (re)negotiating identity through the terrace chant. *Soccer & Society*, *7*, 494–507. https://doi.org/10.1080/14660970600905786

Cross, I. (2006). Four issues in the study of music in evolution. *World Music*, *48*, 233–267.

Drott, E. A. (2018). Music as a technology of surveillance. *Journal of the Society for American Music*, *12*, 233–267.

Dunsworth, H. M., Warrener, A. G., Deacon, T., Ellison, P. T., & Pontzer, H. (2012). Metabolic hypothesis for human altriciality. *Proceedings of the National Academy of Sciences of the United States*, *109*(38),15212–15216. https://doi.org/10.1073/pnas.1205282109

Finnegan, R. (1989) The hidden musicians: Music-making in an English town. Cambridge University Press.

Fleischer, R. (2017). If the song has no price, is it still a commodity? Rethinking the commodification of digital music. *Culture Unbound: Journal of Current Cultural Research*, *9*, 146–162.

Foley, R. A., & Mirazón Lahr, M. (2011). The evolution of the diversity of cultures. *Philosophical Transactions of the Royal Society B: Biological Sciences*, *366*, 1080–1089. https://doi.org/10.1098/rstb.2010.0370

Gould, S. J. (1983). *Hen's teeth and horses' toes*. Penguin.

Harris, I., & Cross, I. (2021). Investigating everyday musical interaction during COVID-19: An experimental procedure for exploring collaborative playlist engagement. *Frontiers in Psychology*, *12*, 1–9. https://doi.org/10.3389/fpsyg.2021.647967

Henrich, J., Heine, S. J., & Norenzayan, A. (2010). Most people are not WEIRD. *Nature*, *466*, 29. https://doi.org/10.1038/466029a

Hesse-Biber, S. (2016). Doing interdisciplinary mixed methods health care research. *Qualitative Health Research*, *26*, 649–658. https://doi.org/10.1177/1049732316634304

Holstein, J. A., & Gubrium, J. F. (2007). Constructionist perspectives on the life course. *Sociology Compass*, *1*, 335–352. https://doi.org/10.1111/j.1751-9020.2007.00004.x

Hove, M. J., & Risen, J. L. (2009). It's all in the timing: Interpersonal synchrony increases affiliation. *Social Cognition*, *27*, 949–961. https://doi.org/10.1521/soco.2009.27.6.949

Katz, M. (2010). *Capturing sound: How technology has changed music*. University of California Press.

Killick, A. (2006). Ethnomusicology forum holicipation: Prolegomenon to an ethnography of solitary music-making. *Ethnomusicology Forum*, *15*, 273–299. https://doi.org/10.1080/17411910600915414

King. G., Currie, M., Smith, L., Servais, M., & McDougall, J. (2008). A framework of operating models for interdisciplinary research programs in clinical service organizations. *Evaluation and Program Planning*, *31*(2), 160–173. https://doi.org/10.1016/j.evalprogplan.2008.01.003

Kohli, M., & Meyer, J. W. (1986). Social structure and social construction of life stages. *Human Development*, *29*, 145–149. https://doi.org/10.1159/000273038

Krumhansl, C. L., & Zupnick, J. A. (2013). Cascading reminiscence bumps in popular music. *Psychological Science*, *24*, 2057–2068. https://doi.org/10.1177/0956797613486486

Kytö, M. (2011). 'We are the rebellious voice of the terraces, we are Çarşı': Constructing a football supporter group through sound. *Soccer & Society*, *12*, 77–93. https://doi.org/10.1080/14660970.2011.530474

Lesko, N. (2012). *Act your age! A cultural construction of adolescence* (2nd ed.). Routledge.

Lewis, J. (2009). As well as words: Congo Pygmy hunting, mimicry, and play. In R. Botha & C. Knight (Eds.), *The cradle of language: Vol. 2. African perspectives* (pp. 381–413). Oxford University Press.

MacLeod, M. (2018). What makes interdisciplinarity difficult? Some consequences of domain specificity in interdisciplinary practice. *Synthese, 195,* 697–720. https://doi.org/10.1007/s11229-016-1236-4

Magee, W. L., Clark, I., Tamplin, J., & Bradt, J. (2017). Music interventions for acquired brain injury. *Cochrane Database of Systematic Reviews.* https://doi.org/10.1002/14651858.CD006787.pub3

Malloch, S., & Trevarthen, C. (2009). *Communicative musicality: Exploring the basis of human companionship.* Oxford University Press.

Mampe, B., Friederici, A., Christophe, A., & Wermke, K. (2009). Newborns' cry melody is shaped by their native language. *Current Biology, 19,* 1994–1997.

Markus, H. R., & Kitayama, S. (2010). Cultures and selves: A cycle of mutual constitution. *Perspectives on Psychological Science, 5,* 420–430. https://doi.org/10.1177/1745691610375557

Merriam, A. P. (1964). *The anthropology of music.* Northwestern University Press.

Nettl, B. (2015). *The study of ethnomusicology: Thirty-three discussions* (3rd ed.). University of Illinois Press.

Nyström, M. E., Karltun, J., Keller, C., & Andersson Gäre, B. (2018). Collaborative and partnership research for improvement of health and social services: Researcher's experiences from 20 projects. *Health Research Policy and Systems, 16,* 46. https://doi.org/10.1186/s12961-018-0322-0

Petticrew, M., & Roberts, H. (2003). Evidence, hierarchies, and typologies: Horses for courses. *Journal of Epidemiology & Community Health, 57,* 527–529. https://doi.org/10.1136/jech.57.7.527

Powell, J., Dosser, D., Handron, D., McCammon, S., Temkin, M. E., & Kaufman, M. (1999). Challenges of interdisciplinary collaboration: A faculty consortium's initial attempts to model collaborative practice. *Journal of Community Practice, 6*(2), 27–48. https://doi.org/10.1300/J125v06n02_03

Rabinowitch, T.-C., Cross, I., & Burnard, P. (2013). Long-term musical group interaction has a positive influence on empathy in children. *Psychology of Music, 41,* 484–498. https://doi.org/10.1177/0305735612440609

Rauscher, F., Shaw, G., & Ky, K. (1993). Music and spatial task performance. *Nature, 365,* 611.

Roseman, M. (2011). A fourfold framework for cross-cultural, integrative research on music and medicine. In B. D. Koen (Ed.), *The Oxford handbook of medical ethnomusicology* (pp. 18–45). Oxford University Press.

Rosenfield, P. L. (1992). The potential of transdisciplinary research for sustaining and extending linkages between the health and social sciences. *Social Science & Medicine, 35,* 1343–1357. https://doi.org/10.1016/0277-9536(92)90038-R

Rudge, A. (2019) Flexibility and egalitarianism: Musical insights from hunter-gatherers. *Ethnomusicology Forum, 28,* 1–21. https://doi.org/10.1080/17411912.2019.1683875

Saarikallio, S., Gold, C., & Mcferran, K. (2015). Development and validation of the Healthy-Unhealthy Music Scale. *Child and Adolescent Mental Health, 20,* 210–217. https://doi.org/10.1111/camh.12109

Sandlana, N. S. (2014). Umoya: Understanding the experiential value of traditional African dance and music for traditional healers. *Mediterranean Journal of Social Sciences, 5,* 541–547. https://doi.org/10.5901/mjss.2014.v5n3p541

Savage, P. E., Loui, P., Tarr, B., Schachner, A., Glowacki, L., Mithen, S., & Fitch, W. (2020). Music as a coevolved system for social bonding. *Behavioral and Brain Sciences, 44,* E59. https://doi.org/10.1017/S0140525X20000333

Schäfer, K., & Eerola, T. (2018). How listening to music and engagement with other media provide a sense of belonging: An exploratory study of social surrogacy. *Psychology of Music, 48,* 232–251. https://doi.org/10.1177/0305735618795036

Schober, M. F., & Spiro, N. (2014). Jazz improvisers' shared understanding: A case study. *Frontiers in Psychology, 5,* 1–21. https://doi.org/10.3389/fpsyg.2014.00808

Silverman, M. J. (2020). Music-based affect regulation and unhealthy music use explain coping strategies in adults with mental health conditions. *Community Mental Health Journal, 56,* 939–946. https://doi.org/10.1007/s10597-020-00560-4

Spiro, N., & Schober, M. F. (2014) Perspectives on music and communication: An introduction. *Psychology of Music, 42,* 771–775. https://doi.org/10.1177/0305735614549493

Spiro, N., & Himberg, T. (2016). Analysing change in music therapy interactions of children with communication difficulties. *Philosophical Transactions of the Royal Society B: Biological Sciences, 371,* 20150374. https://doi.org/10.1098/rstb.2015.0374

Stringer, C. (2016). The origin and evolution of homo sapiens. *Philosophical Transactions of the Royal Society B: Biological Sciences, 371,* 1–12. https://doi.org/10.1098/rstb.2015.0237

Tomasello, M. (1999). The human adaptation for culture. *Annual Review of Anthropology, 28,* 509–529. https://doi.org/10.1146/annurev.anthro.28.1.509

Tomasello, M., & Vaish, A. (2013). Origins of human cooperation and morality. *Annual Review of Psychology, 64,* 231–255. https://doi.org/10.1146/annurev-psych-113011-143812

Trevarthen, C., & Malloch, S. N. (2000). The dance of wellbeing: Defining the musical therapeutic effect. *Nordik Tidsskrift for Musikkterapi, 9*(2), 3–17. https://doi.org/10.1080/08098130009477996

Triandis, H. C., Bontempo, R., Villareal, M. J., Asai, M., & Lucca, N. (1988). Individualism and collectivism: Cross-cultural perspectives on self-ingroup relationships. *Journal of Personality and Social Psychology, 54*(2), 323–338. https://doi.org/10.1037/0022-3514.54.2.323

Tsiris, G., Derrington, P., Sparks, P., Spiro, N., & Wilson, G. (2016). Interdisciplinary dialogues in music, health and wellbeing: Difficulties, challenges and pitfalls. *ISME Commission on Special Education and Music Therapy 2016 proceedings* (pp. 58–70).

Turino. T. (2008) Music as social life: The politics of participation. University of Chicago Press.

Vignoles, V. L., Owe, E., Becker, M., Smith, P. B., Easterbrook, M. J., Brown, R., González, R., Didier, N., Carrasco, D., Cadena, M. P., Lay, S., Schwartz, S. J., Des Rosiers, S. E., Villamar, J. A., Gavreliuc, A., Zinkeng, M., Kreuzbauer, R., Baguma, P., Martin, M., … & Bond, M. H. (2016). Beyond the 'east–west' dichotomy: Global variation in cultural models of self-hood. *Journal of Experiment Psychology: General, 145*(8), 966–1000. https://doi.org/10.1037/xge0000175

Walker, M, (2003) Music as knowledge in shamanism and other healing traditions of Siberia. *Arctic Anthropology, 40,* 40–48.

Name Index

Saarikallio, S., 7, 70–71, 72, 73–74, 75, 76, 77, 91, 152, 153
Sahiner, N. C., 60
Sala, G., 61
Sallnow, L., 121
Salovey, P., 72
Sandlana, N. S., 155
Sanfilippo, K. R. M., 1, 7, 12–13, 15, 19–20, 162
Saunders, C., 120
Savage, P. E., 15, 153
Schäfer, K., 17–18, 157
Schäfer, T., 3
Schellenberg, E. G., 46–49, 50–52, 55–56, 60
Scherer, K., 3
Schetter, C. D., 29
Schlaug, G., 46, 49, 51, 52
Schlez, A., 27
Schmid, W., 133, 137–38, 139
Schober, M. F., 6, 120, 148–49, 150
Schore, A. N., 23
Schroeder-Sheker, T., 123n.3
Schwartz, S. J., 75
Scrine, E., 74–75
Shaffer, D. R., 44, 62
Shahidullah, B. S., 13
Shenfield, T., 16
Shibazaki, K., 132–33
Shin, H. S., 20
Shiner, R. L., 59, 62
Shoemark, H., 25, 27–28, 127
Shonkoff, J. P., 55
Silver, D., 18
Silverman, M. J., 123, 153
Simard, J., 137
Sims, S., 3
Skånland, M. S., 88–89, 90, 135
Skingley, A., 107, 110
Skramstad, H., 18–19
Slivka, H. H., 126
Sloboda, J. A., 3, 45, 47, 59, 70–71, 72, 89–90
Small, C., 3–4, 97
Smoski, W. J., 47–48
Snyder, B., 47
Sole, M., 17
Sonims, V., 24
Speranza, A. M., 20–21
Spiker, D., 24
Spiro, N., 1, 6, 60, 120, 148–49, 150–51
Spychiger, M., 57
Sroufe, L. A., 22
Stacpoole, M., 137
Standley, J. M., 23, 26
Stapleton, M., 73
Stember, M., 138
Stern, D., 73
Stickley, T., 95, 104–5

Stige, B., 95, 133, 139
Stjernswärd, J., 121
Storlien, M., 95
Stringer, C., 156
Stuckler, D., 93
Stultz, S., 22–23, 24
Sung, H.-C., 109
Swaminathan, S., 48, 55–56
Sward, R., 57

Tague, D. B., 123
Tanguay, C. L., 138
Tapson, C., 135
Terry, D. R., 20
Terry, M. M., 20
Theodosius, C., 94
Theorell, T., 55–56
Thomas, L. A., 72
Thompson, R. A., 23
Tomaino, C. M., 57–58
Tomasello, M., 51, 53, 56–57, 60, 156
Toolis, E., 86
Trainor, L. J., 13–14, 15, 16, 21
Trehub, S. E., 7, 12–14, 15, 16–18, 21, 23, 29–30, 44
Trevarthen, C., 22–23, 48–49, 73, 92, 108, 153–54, 156
Triandis, H. C., 156–57
Tsiris, G., 1, 6, 7–8, 119, 119n.1, 120, 123–24, 125–26, 127–28, 128b, 129, 130–31, 133b, 135, 138, 148–49, 162
Tuastad, L., 95
Tudge, J., 46
Tuncgenc, B., 57
Turino, T., 57, 157, 158–59
Turnbull, J., 29

Ueda, T., 109
Uggla, L., 51–52
Ullsten, A., 25, 26

Vaiouli, P., 49, 57–58
Vaish, A., 156
Valentine-French, S., 4
Van Beveren, M. L., 72
van der Heijden, M. J. E., 27
Van Puyvelde, M., 21, 23, 24
Vetter, N. C., 72
Viega, M., 75
Vignoles, V. L., 156–57
Vist, T., 135
Vohs, K. D., 22
Volkova, A., 14

Waage, L., 95
Walker, M., 155

Subject Index

For the benefit of digital users, indexed terms that span two pages (e.g., 52–53) may, on occasion, appear on only one of those pages.

Figures, and boxes are indicated by *f* and *b* following the page number